# Mentoring and Supervision in Healthcare

# Mentoring and Supervision
# in Healthcare

## Neil Gopee

Los Angeles • London • New Delhi • Singapore

First published 2008

Reprinted 2008

 SAGE Publications Ltd
1 Oliver's Yard
55 City Road
London EC1Y 1SP

SAGE Publications Inc.
2455 Teller Road
Thousand Oaks, California 91320

SAGE Publications India Pvt Ltd
B1/I 1 Mohan Cooperative Industrial Area
Mathura Road
New Delhi 110 044

SAGE Publications Asia-Pacific Pte Ltd
33 Pekin Street #02-01
Far East Square
Singapore 048763

Library of Congress Control Number: 2007923184

British Library Cataloguing in Publication data

A catalogue record for this book is available from the
British Library

ISBN 978-1-4129-3019-2
ISBN 978-1-4129-3020-8 (pbk)

Typeset by C&M Digitals (P) Ltd, Chennai, India
Printed in Great Britain by The Cromwell Press Ltd, Trowbridge, Wiltshire
Printed on paper from sustainable resources

# Contents

# List of Boxes, Figures and Tables

## Boxes

## Figures

## Tables

# Acknowledgements

The author of this book would like to acknowledge the support and constructive comments provided by Alison Poyner, Zoë Elliott-Fawcett, Anna Luker and Louise Wise at Sage Publications. I am also thankful to my daughters, Hema, Sheila and Neeta for their support throughout.

This book is also in memory of my father who set high educational standards and aspirations, but passed away in July 2006 while I was still writing this book, as one of my aims of writing was to present him with this book.

Every effort has been made to trace all the copyright holders, but if any have been inadvertently overlooked the publishers will be pleased to make the necessary arrangement at the first opportunity.

Table 1.1
The communication continuum – related purpose and skills, from B. Scammell (1990) *Communication Skills*. Reproduced with permission of Palgrave Macmillan.

Figure 1.2
Diagram on effects of support and challenge on development, in L.A. Daloz (1999) *Mentor: Guiding the Journey of Adult Learners*, page 28. Reproduced with permission of John Wiley and Sons, Inc.

Box 1.4
THE DARLING MMP: MEASURING MENTORING POTENTIAL, IN L.A. DARLING (1985) 'WHAT TO DO ABOUT TOXIC MENTORS?', *JOURNAL OF NURSING ADMINISTRATION*, 14(10): 43. REPRODUCED WITH PERMISSION BY LIPPINCOTT WILLIAMS & WILKINS.

Figure 2.1
D.A. Kolb (1984) *EXPERIENTIAL LEARNING: EXPERIENCE AS A SOURCE OF LEARNING*, PAGE 42. © 1984. ADAPTED WITH THE PERMISSION OF PEARSON EDUCATION, INC., UPPER SADDLE RIVER, NJ.

Box 2.2
A typology of learning, in P. Jarvis and S. Gibson (1997) *The Teacher Practitioner and Mentor Nursing, Midwifery, Health Visiting and the Social Services, second edition*, page 62. Reproduced with permission of Nelson Thornes Ltd.

Table 5.1
A Framework for Practice Development, adapted from S. Page (2001) 'Demystifying practice development', *Nursing Times*, 97(22): 36–7. Reproduced with permission by *Nursing Times*.

Table 6.1
The strengths and weaknesses of self-assessment, in N. Gopee (2000) 'Self-assessment and the concept of the lifelong learning nurse', *British Journal of Nursing*, 9(11): 724–30. Reproduced with permission.

Table 6.2
Advantages and disadvantages of peer-assessment, in N. Gopee (2001) 'The role of peer assessment and peer review in nursing', *British Journal of Nursing*, 10(2): 115–21. Reproduced with permission.

# List of Abbreviations

| | |
|---|---|
| AHP | Allied Health Profession |
| CAIPE | Centre for Advancement of Interprofessional Education |
| CFP | Common foundation programme |
| COPC | Code of Professional Conduct |
| CPD | Continuing professional development |
| DH/DoH | Department of Health |
| EBHC | Evidence-based healthcare |
| EBP | Evidence-based practice |
| ENB | English National Board for Nursing, Midwifery and Health Visiting |
| ESC | Essential skills clusters |
| HEI | Higher Education Institutions |
| HPC | Health Professions Council |
| HTA | Health Technology Assessment |
| IPE | Inter-professional education |
| IPL | Inter-professional learning |
| MMP | Measuring mentorship potential |
| MPE | Multi-professional education |
| NHS III | NHS Institute for Innovation and Improvement |
| *NHS KSF* | *NHS Knowledge and Skills Framework* |
| NMC | Nursing and Midwifery Council |
| OPT | Overhead projector and transparencies |
| OSCE | Objective simulated clinical examination |
| QAA | Quality Assurance Agency for Higher Education |
| RCN | Royal College of Nursing |
| RCT | Randomised controlled trial |
| RM | Registered Midwife |
| RN | Registered Nurse |
| SCPHN | Specialist community public health nurse |
| SDL | Self-directed learning |
| SHA | Strategic Health Authority |
| SLT | Social learning theory |
| STEP | Social, technological, economic and political |
| SWOT | Strengths, weaknesses, opportunities and threats |
| UKCC | United Kingdom Central Council for Nursing, Midwifery and Health Visiting |
| WBL | Work-based learning |

# Introduction

## The Rationale and Scope of this Book

Mentoring has become a significant dimension of professional life (and even personal life), particularly in relation to supporting educational preparation of healthcare professionals. Variously known by different titles such as practice supervisor and clinical educator by different healthcare professions, educational preparation is required for mentors to fulfil this role competently.

Several definitions of this role have evolved over the years, and it was redefined by the English National Board/Department of Health (2001a) following research findings, especially that by Phillips et al. (2000), extending it beyond teaching by mentors to assessment of mentees' clinical competence as well during practice placements. The Nursing and Midwifery Council (NMC) has retained a very similar definition, and in *Standards to Support Learning and Assessment in Practice* (2006a: 14), it identifies 'the underpinning principles for supporting learning and assessment in practice for any student undertaking an NMC approved programme leading to registration or a qualification that is recordable on the register'.

The standards are for registered nurses, registered midwives and specialist community public health nurses (SCPHN) (from here on all healthcare professionals registered with the NMC or the Health Professions Council (HPC) will be referred to as 'registrants'), but they are based on general principles of mentoring or learning supervision so that they are fully applicable to the other three groups of healthcare professions, namely allied health professionals (AHP), social work and medicine. In the current scene of inter-professional learning, reciprocal mentoring between health professions has already been happening at least from the turn of the century.

The NMC standards also identify the criteria for becoming a mentor and make recommendations for preparation programmes (or courses) for mentors. Furthermore, they include details on the roles of practice teachers, the sign-off mentor role, and qualified teacher (e.g. nurse lecturer), along with the competences and outcomes for each of these roles. Continuing professional development and 'monitoring arrangements' are also discussed.

This book addresses the standards, competences and outcomes for mentoring, which is a widely taught topic, and mentorship courses are provided by most universities offering healthcare courses. Furthermore, for a number of reasons, which include the increase in the number of pre-registration nursing students and inter-professional learning, there is an increased demand for mentors, and universities are asked to provide more diverse mentorship education programmes, for example by blended learning.

This book draws on contemporary knowledge on the mechanics of mentoring and aims to enable registrants to acquire the necessary knowledge and skills related to all NMC (2006a) standards for mentors. It thus brings together and builds on existing knowledge of principles and practices of mentoring, and updates it to current-day mentoring requirements. It thus constitutes a firm launchpad for healthcare professionals to further develop and enhance their mentoring expertise.

Recently qualified healthcare professionals who might not yet be functioning in a formal mentoring capacity (associate mentors, for instance) would also find this book useful, as may more experienced qualified health professionals who either haven't completed a mentoring course or who were prepared for the role through a previous 'teaching and assessing' course.

This book is a direct result of my numerous years of experience of teaching and examining on mentoring and 'teaching and assessing' courses, as well as a RN(Registered Nurse) in general and mental health nursing, along with the need for a textbook that reflects current policies and research on mentoring. In addition to current knowledge in the field, this text also recognises the challenges facing both newly qualified and more experienced healthcare professionals whose roles incorporate imparting their clinical knowledge and skills to their juniors and learners quite soon after qualifying, and within resource constraints, role changes, and changing healthcare workforce profiles. It takes into account day-to-day and longer-term issues and challenges in mentoring, and explores potential solutions, where possible supporting them with relevant theories and current research base. The ensuing implications with regard to responsibility and accountability are therefore also explored.

## The Structure of this Book

As just indicated, this book is firmly based on current knowledge in the field, and is structured to ensure that it also addresses all NMC's (2006a) standards for mentors, which also apply to other healthcare professions. Eight 'domains' of competence were initially compiled by the United Kingdom Central Council for Nursing, Midwifery and Health Visiting (UKCC) in 2000, which was revised by the NMC and republished as *A Standard to Support Learning and Assessment in Practice* (2006a). These new standards are detailed under eight revised domains of competences and associated outcomes for mentors, practice teachers and qualified teachers. The final version of this document was published in August 2006 and implemented in mentoring programmes from 2007. This new standard does not identify associate mentors, just NMC registrants, indicating that all registrants have a teaching component in their professional roles. The competences and outcomes are reflected in the choice of content and structure of this textbook.

Each chapter begins by identifying the chapter content under an introduction that includes chapter outcomes, and that is followed by the main text and a chapter summary. A logical combination of text, illustrations, activities, think points, and some case studies is incorporated to engage the reader fully with the material in the book.

Chapter 1 therefore, deals with mentoring as a theme in its own right. It starts by defining the term *mentor*, and differentiates it from other similar or overlapping roles. It thus examines role boundaries between various healthcare learning facilitator roles such as assessors, preceptors and supervisors, as well as practice teachers, and those of link tutors, practice educators and personal tutors. The common aim of all these roles is to facilitate healthcare students and learners to develop clinical competence and knowledge during practice placements.

A number of reasons why mentors are needed for learners on preparatory education programmes in healthcare professions are ascertained, followed by factors that enable the mentoring role to be fulfilled effectively, including the modes of communication needed for effective working relationships between mentors and mentees. Subsequently, the necessary personal and professional attributes of mentors that enable and support the development of learners' clinical skills and knowledge effectively, including being role models, are explored. The nature and detrimental effects of poor or adverse mentoring are also discussed, followed by an examination of different models of effective mentoring.

Having identified the crucial role that mentoring occupies in enabling learning in clinical settings, Chapter 2 takes a detailed look at how learning occurs. It examines major perspectives on learning, and learning theories, styles and approaches. Chapter 3 builds on this and explores facilitation of learning. The chapter starts by ascertaining the range of people whom healthcare professionals teach, followed by the reasons for teaching and learning. It then focuses on how healthcare students learn patient or service-user care delivery skills in clinical settings, and how the mentor utilises opportunities for informal teaching.

The concept of facilitation of learning, as distinct from teaching, is examined, followed by key perceptions and major views, approaches and styles of teaching including andragogy. The levels and stages of skill acquisition (taxonomy levels) are explored, and the types of knowledge associated with skills, for example practical knowledge and theoretical knowledge, are considered, along with levels of theory acquisition.

This is closely followed by steps in lesson planning for structured short teaching sessions for teaching skills and knowledge on a one-to-one level, or for teaching small groups of learners or peers. The chapter then discusses different teaching or presentation methods and the use of different teaching aids. A discussion follows on some of the more common difficulties that mentors might encounter when undertaking short structured teaching sessions, and the likely solutions for them.

Following on from facilitation of learning, Chapter 4 focuses on the attributes that make clinical settings effective learning environments, which is a key component of the mentor role (Darling, 1984; NMC, 2006a). The NMC indicates that the mentor should create and develop opportunities for students to identify and undertake experiences to meet their learning needs. Students' perspectives on practice placements, such as their own expectations and their practice objectives, are considered, followed by an examination of the part played by national guidelines and current policy documents on practice placements. Issues related to practice placements are also examined.

Research on clinical learning environments, which underpins the development of the tool for annual educational audits of practice placement areas, is then examined. Educational audits include identifying learning resources (human and material) that are available in clinical settings, inter-professional learning, and how the clinical area can become, or form part of, a learning organization. The utilisation of learning pathways (based on patient journeys), which can be incorporated in learning contracts, can play an important role in ensuring the success of the placement. Finally, work-based learning is also examined.

Fundamental to mentorship are evidence-based practice (EBP), research implementation, clinical practice development and management of change. These constitute the focus of Chapter 5. Research by Darling (1984), for instance, and the NMC (2006a) standards for mentorship firmly indicate that the role of the mentor incorporates full awareness and close monitoring by the mentor of their own standards of patient or service-user care.

It is incumbent upon the mentor, as a role model for mentees, to practise evidence-based care, which mentors can do by utilising sources of evidence such as electronic databases where critically appraised evidence is stored. Critical evaluation of research evidence is discussed, including levels or grades of evidence. The concept of clinical practice development, and how the mentor achieves this, is explored in detail, as is the mentor's role in identifying, evaluating, disseminating and applying research findings, and the implementation and management of change.

One of the principal purposes of mentoring programmes is to equip course attendees with the capability to assess students' clinical competencies. Ongoing assessment of competence of healthcare practitioners is a fundamental component of the mentor role and therefore of all course programmes for skill-based healthcare professions, and this is the area that Chapter 6 focuses on.

To fulfil this key mentor function effectively, the mentor needs to know and understand the principles and processes of assessment, that is, why assess, what assessments are and who performs them, and when and how they are conducted. As to what assessments are, various definitions of assessment are considered, followed by the specific aims of assessments. Student self-assessment and peer assessment are also examined.

Under how to assess, the chapter explores key principles of assessments, including dimensions of assessment, as well as levels and fairness of assessments. Other crucial attributes of assessments are their validity and reliability, which are also explored in some detail, the aim being to ascertain the assessee's fitness to practise. Furthermore, the role of policies and procedures in the management of assessments is explored, along with giving feedback and documentation of assessments.

Before assessing the learner's competencies, the mentor needs to plan a placement learning programme carefully for the mentee and have a good understanding of how to assess and implement approved assessment procedures. Recent research findings have highlighted various day-to-day problems encountered by both mentors and students related to the assessment of competence during clinical placements. Therefore the mentor needs to exercise leadership, which includes forward planning to avert problems of assessment. Chapter 7 delves into the details of various potential problems that could occur with assessments, such as those detailed by Phillips et al. (2000), and how they should be prevented or resolved, and includes ethical and legal aspects of mentoring.

The mentor's accountability, responsibility and the use of 'professional judgement' are examined in the context of the mentor's leadership role. Supporting the student, who is generally perceived as struggling to progress with their placement learning, is also examined, including the role of action planning and reassessment of the learner. Intra- and inter-mentor reliability is also explored.

The facilitation of learning and assessment of learners' competence are therefore essential components of the mentor role. Chapter 8 concentrates on the evaluation of teaching and assessment. The nature and purpose of evaluation amount to the mentor self-monitoring the quality of their mentoring. The chapter therefore considers what evaluation is, who is involved in the evaluation of learning facilitation and assessment, and how they are performed, including the use of models of evaluation. The challenges of facilitation of learning and assessment are examined, followed by an examination of the mentor's ongoing professional development, incorporating an overview of continuing professional development and lifelong learning.

## How to Use this Book

This book examines the knowledge base, skills and attitudes required for mentoring, and the NMC's standards for mentors. The text explores theories and research on mentoring, analyses their strengths and weaknesses and examines how they can be applied to day-to-day mentoring and clinical practice activities.

This textbook adopts an analytical and interactive style, with a clear focus on the means of application of theories and principles to various clinical settings. Therefore, throughout the book, the reader is encouraged, through activities and think points, to explore and apply concepts to their practice and roles. The activities usually ask the reader to consider a particular point or component and make some notes, while think points ask the reader to reflect on their own experience and knowledge, prior to moving on with the text. Consequently, the reader needs to interact with the text to achieve optimum benefit. It also allows mentors to exercise freedom and scope to be creative in enabling and facilitating mentees' learning.

A few mini case studies are incorporated as examples of situations that the mentor might encounter, with the aim of exploring how the mentor can approach them for effective mentoring and assessing. Furthermore, some of the boxes (e.g. Box 4.1) are derived from a number of workshops on mentor preparation programmes. As events evolve and different clinical settings have their own specific characteristics, feel free to note other components you can add to the content of these boxes.

The term *healthcare professionals* is used in the text to signify all healthcare employees, medical and non-medical, including nurses and allied health professionals, who hold a qualification that is recognized by either their national regulatory body or professional body. The term *registrant* refers to healthcare professionals on either the NMC or HPC professional registers. The term *learner* is used to refer to everyone who wants or needs to learn healthcare skills, while *students* are those learners who are actually following a professional course leading to a university qualification.

# ONE

# Effective Mentoring

## Introduction

The first chapter of this book examines the concept of mentoring itself, along with the activities associated with it. It draws on a wide range of perspectives on mentoring, and covers:

- The concept of mentoring, its origins, the current range of perceptions and use of the term, and related learning-facilitation functions in various settings and educational programmes.
- The reasons for learners needing mentors and the criteria that need to be fulfilled to be able to use the title of mentor.
- Effective mentoring, which comprises the characteristics of mentors that enable, and the actions that support learning, including building sound mentor–mentee 'working' relationships.
- The adverse effects of poor mentoring.
- Models and guidelines for effective mentoring.

The chapter explores a wide range of perspectives on mentoring, which include the relevant NMC's (2006a: 48) mentor competence: 'Demonstrate effective relationship building skills sufficient to support learning, as part of a wider interprofessional team, for a range of students in both practice and academic learning environments.' The NMC's outcomes for this competence are:

- Develop effective working relationships based on mutual trust and respect.
- Demonstrate an understanding of factors that influence how students integrate into practice settings.
- Provide ongoing and constructive support to facilitate transition from one learning environment to another.

### Chapter outcomes

On completion of this chapter you should be able to:

1. Distinguish between mentoring and similar roles in supporting professional learning.
2. Explain a range of reasons why mentors are required for enabling learners to gain professional knowledge and competence.

3. Identify and evaluate a number of factors that could enable effective mentoring.
4. Analyse the effects of inefficient or adverse mentoring.
5. Critically analyse a range of approaches and models that are used to enable more systematic mentoring.

## The Concept of Mentoring

Mentoring as a concept and practice that is related to facilitating professional learning in healthcare has evolved consistently since the 1970s and was formally implemented in the 1980s. Slightly different titles and terminologies are used by different healthcare professional groups for this role, and different definitions have been offered over time as research and expert opinions have influenced the form in which it is currently utilised.

It is generally well documented, for example in the *Shorter Oxford English Dictionary* (Brown, 2002: 1747), that the term 'mentor' originates from the Greek classic story, *The Odyssey*, in which King Odysseus calls upon a trusted friend named Mentor to act as the guide and advisor to his son Telemachus while he goes to another country to fight a war. The word mentor also relates to the Latin word '*mens*' that is, pertaining to, or occurring in the mind (Simpson and Weiner, 1989: 614). The term has gradually evolved to signify a designated person who takes time out to help people to learn during their developmental years, to progress towards and achieve maturity and establish their identity. It has been implemented as a formal role in nurse education to direct focus on enabling learners to gain clinical skills during practice placements. This section disentangles the concept of mentor from similar titles by exploring the differences and similarities between them.

### Distinguishing between the mentor's and related roles

### Activity 1.1 – Different education support roles and functions

To begin with, make notes on what you think are the meanings and functions of the roles of mentor, preceptor, clinical supervisor, assessor and other similar ones you have encountered, and the differences between them.

*Mentor*
Beside the helping function during developmental years indicated by dictionary definitions of the term *mentor*, as a result of research by Phillips et al. (2000) on behalf of the then English National Board for Nursing, Midwifery and Health Visiting (ENB) and the Department of Health (DH) (2001a), mentor was redefined as a nurse, midwife or health visitor who facilitates learning, supervises and assesses students in

the clinical setting. Prior to this, the mentor was a registrant who facilitated learning, and the assessor was another registrant who assessed learners' competencies.

It is defined similarly by the NMC (2006a) as a registrant who has met the outcomes of Stage 2 (i.e. those of a qualified mentor) and who facilitates learning, and supervises and assesses students in a practice setting. The ENB/DH's (2001a) definition resulted from a range of issues related to mentoring and assessing pre-registration students during clinical placements revealed by Phillips et al.'s (2000) research and other studies earlier on (e.g. White et al. 1993).

Before this, the ENB (1997: 37) had defined a mentor as a 'first level nurse/midwife/health visitor who, by example and facilitation, guides, assists and supports the student's learning … has an understanding of the context of the student's learning experience and is selected by the student'. The notion that students can select their mentor has currency in some situations, despite the problems of mentoring highlighted by Phillips et al. (2000). However, Spouse (2001a) found that the terms *mentorship, preceptorship* and *supervision* were being used synonymously, while White et al. (1993) had earlier found that mentors themselves were unclear about their roles due to lack of educational preparation. However, Kerry and Mayes (1995) note that definitions of mentor need to include:

- nurturing;
- role modeling;
- functioning (as teacher, sponsor, encourager, counsellor and friend);
- focusing on the professional development of the mentee; and
- sustaining a caring relationship over time.

### Preceptor

As the term most closely related to mentor, the NMC identifies *preceptors* as first-level registrants who have had at least 12 months' (or equivalent) experience within the same area of practice as the practitioner requiring support: 'They … should be able to demonstrate a willingness and aptitude for the role … and must be keen to share their knowledge … and appreciate the additional demands it will place upon them' (NMC, 2006b: 1). The NMC indicates that the preceptor and the practitioner requiring support should agree on the nature of their working relationship and define desired outcomes as appropriate.

The preceptor role emerged from the realisation that for newly qualified nurses going from being a student to becoming a registered healthcare professional is a major transition. It is based on an earlier study by Kramer (1974) who found that the first few months after qualifying were often marked by dramatically conflicting value systems, between the aims of pre-registration education and the reality of day-to-day nursing. This led to high attrition rates among newly qualified nurses. Various studies reveal such concerns even today.

The NMC (2006c) recommends preceptorship for all new registrants, that is, for newly qualified registrants, for nurses returning to practice after a break of five years or more, for RNs changing their area of practice, and for qualified nurses from other European Economic Area states and overseas. It indicates that for preceptorship to be effective, new registrants should have a period of preceptorship of approximately four months, and complete a mentor or practice teacher preparation programme. The NMC's (2006c) recommendations for the preceptor role are as follows. The preceptor should:

- Facilitate the transition of the 'new registrant' from student to a registrant who is confident in their practice, sensitive to the needs of patients/clients, an effective team member and up to date with their practice and knowledge.
- Provide feedback to 'new registrants' on those aspects of performance that are being undertaken well.
- Provide honest and objective feedback on those aspects of performance that are a cause for concern and assist 'new registrants' to develop a plan of action to remedy these.
- Facilitate new registrants to gain new knowledge and skills.
- Be aware of the standards, competencies or objectives set by the employer that the 'new registrant' is required to achieve, and support them in achieving these.

Structured preceptorship programmes are devised locally by trusts or clinical settings and are normally of four to six months' duration, and often include the specialism-specific competencies in the induction programmes for the particular clinical setting, which the preceptee can subsequently incorporate in their professional portfolio. The NMC (2006d) notes that the qualities of a willing and able preceptor include knowledge of pre-registration curriculum, leadership skills, ability to act as a role model, interest/aptitude in role, level of experience, awareness of confidentiality and approachability.

### Assessor

The term 'assessor' remains in use and is often used to denote a role similar to that of the mentor but with a definite assessment component (ENB/DH, 2001a). Previously, the ENB (1997: 36) had indicated that the assessor is an 'appropriately qualified and experienced first level nurse/midwife/health visitor who has undertaken preparation and annual updating to develop skills in facilitating student learning, supervising practice and assessing the student's level of attainment related to the stated learning outcomes of the programme'.

### Clinical educator

This is a role akin to mentoring and is generally used by some healthcare professions such as medicine and physiotherapy for student learning during practice placements.

### Clinical supervision

Clinical supervision refers to a peer-support role based on a clinically focused professional relationship between the healthcare professional and a clinical supervisor. The clinical supervisor undergoes educational preparation for this role and utilises clinical knowledge and experience to assist peers to further develop their own knowledge, competence, values and practices.

*Clinical supervisor*
A term used in the context of clinical supervision signifying the provider of peer support to the clinical supervisee. It may be used to identify mentoring-type roles in some healthcare professions or vocations.

*Practice teacher*
This title or role was initially specifically adopted in recognition of the additional preparation required for mentoring students on SCPHN courses. A practice teacher is 'a registrant who normally will have previously fulfilled the NMC requirements to become a mentor, and who has received further preparation to achieve the knowledge, skills and competence required to meet the NMC defined outcomes for a practice teacher' (NMC, 2006a: 20). It refers to specialist areas of practice where they support students undertaking a specialist qualification or at a level beyond initial registration.
    Practice teaching, practice learning and student supervision are terms that are also used for mentoring student social workers during practice placements (Shardlow and Doel, 1996).

*Registrant*
A nurse, midwife or allied health professional currently on the NMC or HPC registers. The NMC (2006a) clearly specifies that all registrants have a teaching role towards others in the clinical setting.

*Supervision*
In healthcare, the term *supervision* is used in counselling situations whereby one or more highly experienced counsellors help a colleague or more junior counsellor develop their practice. The British Association for Counselling and Psychotherapy (2006: 4) defines supervision as 'the reflexive exploration and development of helping practice, in a supportive yet challenging context, involving individuals in the role(s) of supervisee and supervisor'.

*Supervisor*
The term *supervisor* tends to be used in the context of management of workers to ensure designated tasks are completed, rather than in relation to facilitation of learning. It is defined as 'any individual having authority in the interest of the employer to hire, transfer, suspend, lay off, recall, promote, discharge, assign, reward, or discipline other employees' (Sullivan and Decker, 2005: 362).
    Other learning facilitation support roles that are similar to the mentor's have been identified by various agents, some of which are still at nascent stages, and include practice facilitator, buddy, coach, and co-tutor.

## Roles of practice educators, personal tutors and link tutors

The roles of facilitators of learning who are fully or partly employed by universities include practice educator, personal tutor and link tutor.

*Practice educator*

The practice educator role in nursing and midwifery also emerged largely from the study of mentors by Phillips et al. (2000). It is defined as a 'role of the teacher of nursing, midwifery or health visiting who makes a significant contribution to education in the practice setting, co-ordinating student experiences and assessment of learning' (ENB/DH, 2001a: 6). The practice educator leads the development of practice and provides support and guidance to mentors and others who contribute to the student's experience in practice, enabling them to meet learning outcomes and develop appropriate competencies.

The educational preparation for the practice educator role is at post-graduate level. The post is generally funded directly by Strategic Health Authorities and entails practice-based teaching four days a week and university-based teaching one day. This is a very important role as practice educators are also called upon to work with students during practice placements when busy clinical staff are unable to dedicate sufficient extra attention to students who are struggling or failing to progress with their practice placement competencies.

For AHPs, the Society of Radiographers, for instance, adopts the Higher Education Academy (2005: 7) definition of practice educator, which is: 'the identified practitioner in practice placement who facilitates student learning face to face on a daily basis and generally has responsibility for the formative and/or summative assessment'. The preparation of AHPs' practice educators is somewhat similar to the mentor role in nursing and midwifery, and can take either the experiential route or a taught programme of six days' workshops spread over several months – see HPC, College of Occupational Therapists or Chartered Society of Physiotherapy websites for details.

*Personal tutor*

Each pre-registration student is allocated to a nurse lecturer who acts as a personal tutor to the student. This role normally lasts for the duration of the three-year pre-registration course, and involves:

- Supporting, advising and monitoring students' progress throughout the educational programme.
- Accessing students' practice records, within an ethos of confidentiality and professional accountability.
- Liaising with the mentor, link tutor and student and, where concern is expressed, considering evidence and developing an action plan with the student.

*Link tutor*

The link tutor is usually a university lecturer whose responsibility is to assist clinicians in named clinical settings. They assist mentors to interpret students' practice competencies and are available to support mentors when required. They might also assist in the development of the clinical setting as a more effective learning environment for all learners. Students tend to receive a visit by the link tutor early in the allocation, to ascertain which learning objectives are realistically achievable. Further visits are arranged as required.

Some of the functions of the personal tutor and the link tutor have increasingly become part of the practice educator's remit but they continue to provide an essential complementary function.

## Why Do Learners Need Mentors?

The mentor role is widely implemented and utilised and it may now appear to be an obvious facility afforded to learners. A more detailed examination of why we need mentors for mentoring students and learners reveals a number of reasons.

### Activity 1.2 – Why mentors?

The idea of this activity is to explore the variety of reasons why mentors are required in healthcare professional education, particularly in the context of the prevailing definition of the term. Therefore, consider and make notes on the question, 'Why do we need mentors (and preceptors) in (a) nursing, midwifery and allied health professions; and (b) personal life. List as many reasons as you can think of.

When students on mentoring courses are asked to cite as many reasons as they can think of for requiring mentors, they tend to be able to identify several of these. The reasons given include the need to ensure safe practice by learners, to enable students to achieve their course practice competencies, and to listen and act as a sounding board for any worries or fears, or the mentee's ideas on care delivery. Further reasons cited by students for mentoring learners in (a) nursing, midwifery, and allied health professions; and (b) personal life are listed in Box 1.1.

---

**Box 1.1   Why we need mentors**

*In nursing and other health professions*

- For guidance and support
- To structure working environment for learning
- For constructive and honest feedback
- For debriefing related to good/bad experience during placement
- As a link person with other areas
- As role model
- To assess competence
- As a friend and counsellor
- For seeking answers to questions
- For protection from poor practice
- To build confidence
- For sharing learning, i.e. learning from each other
- It is a NMC requirement
- To keep own skills and knowledge up to date
- For linking theory to practice

---

*(Continued)*

- For encouragement
- To provide the appropriate knowledge base for nursing interventions

- For developing one's work role
- To provide structured learning programmes during practice placements

*In personal life*

- For development of one's self
- To share experiences
- For encouragement
- To build confidence

- For honest opinions and views
- As role model (may be parent figure, etc.)
- For socialisation
- For support and guidance

It could be argued that everyone could benefit from having a 'mentor', at times referred to as a 'soulmate'. This privileged role is self-selected by both parties and could be filled by a friend, partner, parent or senior peer. It is consistent with the ENB's (1997) previous definition of mentor, which suggested that the mentor is selected by the learner for support and guidance. Student mentors identify various reasons for the mentoring role. There are also various research and policy reasons for instituting this role. The most significant ones for healthcare are now discussed.

First, mentoring has been implemented quite effectively in non-healthcare professions and social contexts. For instance, mentoring has worked successfully in initial teacher training (Furlong and Maynard, 1995; Kerry and Mayes, 1995) for some time. Mentoring has also become an increasingly popular concept in a wide range of settings, for example:

- in schools and other educational institutions – to raise achievement, self-confidence, personal and social skills;
- in business – to support personal development of business skills, human resource strategies, and business development and self-employment;
- in support of young people who are, or are at risk of becoming, disaffected or excluded from society.

Second, when nurse education moved into the higher education sector *en masse* during the 1980s and 1990s with the restructured Project 2000 pre-registration curricula and a change in emphasis in certain aspects, the findings of various pieces of research on these novel programmes were captured eventually in the UKCC's *Fitness for Practice* (1999) publication. It documented the strengths of these programmes, but one of the prominent findings of these studies was that at the point of registration students were not clinically as skilled as those who emerged from pre-Project 2000 programmes. This reinforced the need for wider availability of competent clinically based mentors to enable students to learn clinical skills and become 'fit for practice'.

**Figure 1.1   The four processes of learning**

The *Dearing Report* on learning in higher education, and other related national reports, also strongly advocate that higher education courses should enable students to become fit for practice, fit for purpose and fit for award (National Committee for Inquiry into Higher Education, 1997).

Third, the findings of Kramer's (1974) study mentioned earlier indicated the need for preceptors for newly qualified nurses. The notion was extrapolated to pre-registration students and is also a reason for the introduction of the term mentor in the UK in the 1980s as a means of supporting student nurses with their learning during practice placements.

Fourth, the 'standards or codes of professional conduct' for nurses, doctors, social workers and AHPs usually indicate that qualified practitioners have a duty to facilitate learners to develop their competence (e.g. NMC, 2004a: clause 6.4). Similar requirements feature in healthcare practitioners' job descriptions, which are also guided by the *NHS Knowledge and Skills Framework (NHS KSF)* (DH, 2004a).

Mentoring of course also provides registrants with an opportunity to teach, which in itself is a feature of their own professional development and can act as a stepping stone in their own career paths.

Finally, another reason for mentoring is the concept of work-based learning, which constitutes practice-based development of skills and (practical) knowledge. Its main features are reflected in the social learning theory which was constituted by Bandura (1977, 1986) and centres on learning skills by observing skilled professionals perform them first. Social learning theory therefore also involves mentors being role models, and comprises four processes of learning (Figure 1.1):

In more detail, the four processes of learning that the learner goes through are:

1.  *Observation of skilled performance*
    (a)   individual observes a skilled performance ('modelling stimulus');
    (b)   the observed behaviour is seen as useful and distinctive;
    (c)   observer's level of arousal pertaining to the skill is raised;

(d)  observer is keen to learn the skill;

(e)  observer has previously felt positive reinforcement for learning skills.

2.  *Mental retention of the skill*

(a)  step-by-step performance of the skill is mentally assimilated;

(b)  mental rehearsal of modelled behaviour.

3.  *Motor reproduction of the skill*

(a)  Observer carries out observed behaviour or skill, and self-evaluates it in terms of performance.

4.  *Reinforcement and adoption*

(a)  The behaviour is reinforced by external reward such as praise or through self-reinforcement and is likely to be adopted.

According to Bandura (1977), we do not possess any inherent behaviour patterns at birth except reflexes, and therefore learning occurs by observing other people, which is the essence of social learning theory and which therefore includes learning from social situations. In healthcare, learners (mentees and preceptees) learn and acquire practical skills from mentors and other healthcare professionals through the four processes identified in Figure 1.1.

Bandura's (1977) social learning theory had previously been termed observational learning or modelling, and was built on behaviourist learning theory (see Chapter 2). It is a component of work-based learning, which is examined in detail in Chapter 4 in the context of learning in clinical settings.

## Who Can Be a Mentor?

Despite all the reasons for mentoring discussed so far, it shouldn't be taken for granted that all qualified healthcare professionals wish to undertake mentoring work some or all of the time. Some healthcare professionals feel that continuous allocation of students to them all year round can be detrimental to their own effectiveness with their workloads, and they would like some space for reflection and to focus on their own professional development.

In the selection of mentors, it is important to ensure they have the necessary skills and expertise for mentoring, which according to Neary (2000a) include coaching, counselling, facilitating, setting standards, assessing and giving feedback. Other writers and researchers identify similar lists of skills. Such lists initially appear simplistic as a whole range of expertise is required to undertake the mentorship role, and this can be developed only through appropriate educational preparation.

The ENB's (1997) guidelines suggested that students should be able to select their mentor in each placement but in reality this is difficult in many clinical settings due to various factors such as RNs' increased workload. Others may select one individual to whom they can relate throughout the entire programme as a personal mentor or a 'buddy'. Furthermore, the NMC (2006a) also identifies the criteria for who can be mentors for nursing and midwifery learners, which are as follows:

- Be registered in the same part or sub-part of the register as the student they are to assess and, for the nurses' part of the register, be in the same field of practice (adult, mental health, learning disability or children's).
- Have developed their own knowledge, skills and competence beyond registration, that is, have been registered for at least one year.
- Have successfully completed an NMC-approved mentor preparation programme (or a comparable programme which has been accredited by an AEI – Approved Education Institution – as meeting the NMC mentor requirements).
- Have the ability to select, support and assess a range of learning opportunities in their area of practice for students undertaking NMC-approved programmes.
- Be able to support learning in an inter-professional environment – selecting and supporting a range of learning opportunities for students from other professions.
- Have the ability to contribute to the assessment of other professionals under the supervision of an experienced assessor from that profession.
- Be able to make judgements about competence/proficiency of NMC students on the same part of the register, and in the same field of practice, and be accountable for such decisions.
- Be able to support other registrants in meeting CPD (continuing professional development) needs in accordance with *The NMC Code of Professional Conduct: Standards for Conduct, Performance and Ethics (NMC, 2004a)*.

These criteria clearly imply that not all registrants are suitable for mentoring, at least not for all categories of learners. The competencies and outcomes for mentors are discussed shortly.

## Effective Mentoring

The principles and methods of mentoring incorporate a number of factors that are essential for effective student learning. They include meeting NMC's (2006a) standards for mentors identified under eight domains, these being:

1. establishing effective working relationships;
2. facilitation of learning;
3. assessment and accountability;
4. evaluation of learning;
5. creating an environment for learning;
6. context of practice;
7. evidence-based practice;
8. leadership.

The first domain, 'establishing effective working relationships', encompasses:

- how effective working relationships are developed and maintained;
- effective mentor–mentee communication;
- characteristics of the mentor;
- actions by mentor that support learning, including the use of learning contracts.

Each of the other domains is addressed separately in subsequent chapters as detailed in the introduction to this book.

## Effective working relationships

For two individuals who are usually initially unknown to each other, adopting the mentor–mentee roles presupposes that they have to be able to communicate with each other, develop a rapport, and cultivate a 'working' relationship at the very least. The word *rapport* means 'a state of deep spiritual, emotional or mental connection between people', including understanding and empathy (Brown, 2002: 2465), and *relationship* refers to 'the state or fact of being related, an emotional association between two people' (Brown, 2002: 2520). The requirement for effective working relationships is recognised by the NMC (2006a). But how are relationships formed between two designated parties? According to Rogers and Freiberg (1994), counsellors and helpers build a trusting and working relationship by first of all ensuring that certain key conditions prevail. These are:

- Acceptance – (or unconditional positive regard) of the individual for who they are, that is, for their individual strengths and weaknesses, and mutual respect.
- Genuineness – as a person, honesty.
- Empathic understanding – being able and willing to view situations from the other person's perspective.

These key conditions are explored in some detail in the context of student-centred learning in Chapter 3. Rogers and Freiberg (1994) emphasise that 'trust' underpins these key conditions, which, they suggest in reality permeate all mutually beneficial relationships. It is akin to a 'psychological contract' between the mentor and mentee, or between patient and carer, colleagues and friends. The two parties also have to be willing to spend time together to maintain this relationship, and to work towards the achievement of practice objectives, for instance. Although the mentee has to actively seek out relevant learning opportunities, the mentor also needs to take actions that support the mentee's learning, for example by familiarising themselves adequately with the mentee's educational programme.

## Effective mentor–mentee communication

The skills and techniques of communication are some of the most important tools the practitioner undertaking the mentoring role has to utilise. The healthcare professional is normally already a skilled communicator through initial educational preparation, and therefore it is important to establish which other communication techniques they need to develop to extend their skillbase. Effective communication skills are essential within all teaching and learning situations. So what is communication?

The word 'communication' originates from the Latin word '*communicare*' which means to impart, share, convey or exchange information (Brown, 2002: 463). It is 'a complex, ongoing dynamic process in which the participants simultaneously create shared meaning in an interaction. The goal of communication is to approach, as closely as possible, a common understanding of the message sent, and the one received' (Sullivan and Decker, 2005: 123). The factors influencing communication are:

- past conditioning;
- the present situation;
- each person's purpose in the communication;
- each person's attitudes towards self, the topic, and each other.

Various modes of communication are available to the mentor to choose from, including:

- Written, for example handwritten, typed, emailed, faxed, printed.
- Oral (spoken), for example face to face, one to one, in groups, by telephone.
- Non-verbal, for example body posture, eye contact, tone of voice.

Oral (spoken) communication is always accompanied by non-verbal messages, vocal and non-vocal. In fact non-verbal hues are more powerful than verbal messages. Furthermore Argyle (1994) suggests that non-verbal signals of a friendly attitude (as opposed an unfriendly attitude) are:

- *Proximity*: closer, leaning forward if seated.
- *Orientation*: more direct, but side to side for some situations.
- *Gaze*: more gaze, and mutual gaze.
- *Facial expression*: more smiling.
- *Gestures*: head nods, lively movements.
- *Posture*: open arms stretched towards each other rather than arms on hips or folded.
- *Touch*: more touch in an appropriate manner.
- *Tone of voice*: higher pitch, upward contour, pure tone.
- *Verbal contents*: more self-disclosure.

The normal communication process is often presented as the information processing theory in the context of cognitive learning theory, which is discussed in Chapter 2.

*Generic and specialist communication skills*
In addition to general communication skills, the mentor is likely to need to develop specialist communication skills to deal with emerging mentoring situations. Scammell (1990) suggests a communication continuum of generic to specialist communication, the related skills and who uses them (see Table 1.1).

Primary and secondary communication occurs between mentor and mentee when exchanging information and establishing a working relationship. Beyond this level, the mentor may need to give direct advice to the student, especially when teaching, as well as when advice is requested. This however does not go as far as counselling, for which the individual requires more extensive training.

Primary counselling is a specialised communication skill that the mentor needs to develop to deal with difficult mentoring situations. Secondary counselling will be required for more intense psychological problems, which the mentor can deal with by directing the student to appropriate support services, or, if trained, by using a systematic approach such as Heron's (1989) six-category intervention analysis (see Box 1.2).

**Table 1.1   The communication continuum – related purpose and skills**

|  | Primary communications | Secondary communications | Advice giving | Primary counselling | Secondary counselling |
|---|---|---|---|---|---|
| *Purpose* | Initial contacts with others; brief encounters | Ongoing relationships – verbal, non-verbal, written; informal support groups | To offer factual information; to teach, instruct, supervise | Support for friend or work colleague | Therapeutic counselling for specific mental health problems |
| *Skills and knowledge needed* | Simple interpersonal or social skills, e.g. ability to listen, etc. | Interpersonal or social skills, knowledge of how groups work, etc. | When to give advice, knowledge of subject, etc. | Listen non-judgementally, help with problem-solving, etc. | Advanced accurate empathy, self-disclosure, etc. |

*Source*: Scammell (1990).

---

Box 1.2   The six-category intervention analysis as a specialised communication skill

*Authoritative intervention*

- Prescriptive: giving advice
- Informative: imparting information
- Confrontational: directly challenging

*Facilitative intervention*

- Supportive: understanding and encouraging
- Cathartic: allowing the release of emotions
- Catalytic: encouraging deeper exploration

---

Heron's (1989) six-category intervention analysis entails six possible actions that the counsellor can choose from. In difficult mentor–mentee situations, for every interaction, the mentor may decide which of the six categories is most appropriate. For instance, for a student who frequently claims to be feeling unwell, physically or psychologically, the mentor might use the prescriptive category of helping, and advise the mentee to consult the occupational health department. They might also give further information about where the department is, and the likely outcomes of this situation. In other situations, the mentor might use another one of the categories, for example cathartic, to enable the mentee to elaborate in detail how they feel about a patient whom they have looked after but who has passed away rather suddenly.

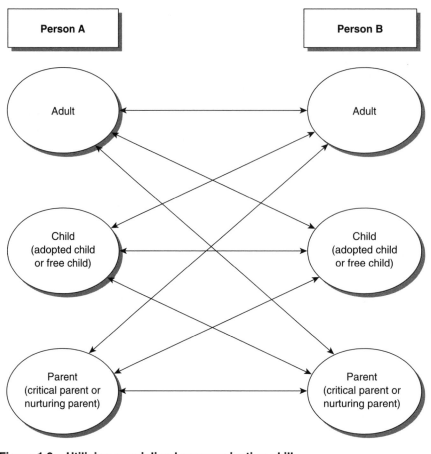

**Figure 1.2 Utilising specialised communication skill: transactional analysis**

Another specialised communication skill involves communicating in one of three ways, or from one of three ego states (how we act, feel and behave) (Berne, 1975). It is known as transactional analysis, and illustrated in Figure 1.2.

In transactional analysis, every item of communication is uttered from one of the three ego states and received from one of the three ego states. Resolution of the inter-personal or psychological problem is achieved when both individuals communicate from adult ego states.

Transactional analysis is also a therapeutic technique that normally requires formal training. To extend communication skills to the arena of assessment of practice objectives, the mentor could find that they have to utilise specialised communication skill in helping and counselling the student who fails an assessment. This would entail aspects of counselling and helping skills that are relevant for the particular assessment situation.

Characteristics of mentors and enabling
functions

## Activity 1.3 – Characteristics of an effective mentor

Make a list of what you consider to be the characteristics of a registrant who is effective in their mentoring role for either pre- or post-registration students. Consider their characteristics from such perspectives as personal qualities, approach/actions and skills.

Responding to Activity 1.3 must have been straightforward as all healthcare professionals who have undertaken preparatory educational programmes that include practice placement will have encountered mentors. Some mentors may have been excellent, while there might have been reservations about others. Most of the characteristics identified by groups of student mentors are listed in Box 1.3.

---

**Box 1.3   Characteristics of the person who needs to act as mentor**

- Patient
- Open-minded
- Approachable
- Has a good knowledge base
- Knowledge and competence is up to date
- Has good communication skills, including listening skills
- Provides encouragement
- Self-motivated
- Shows concern, compassion, empathy
- Has teaching skills
- Provides psychological support
- Counsellor

- Tactful
- Diplomatic, fun and fair
- Willing to be a mentor
- Versatile, adaptable, flexible
- Allows time and commits self to it
- Confident
- Enthusiastic
- Advisor
- Honest and trustworthy
- Trusting
- A role model
- Non-judgemental
- Resource facilitator
- Able to build working relationship

---

Darling (1984) reports on a study that explored various components of the mentor role. One of the most significant outcomes of the study was the identification of the characteristics of mentors that enable learning, as detailed in Box 1.4.

Each mentor characteristic can be explored in detail as a concept in its own right, and to illustrate this the next section explores the characteristic of 'role model' and then of 'challenger and supporter'.

## Box 1.4  Characteristics and roles of mentors

| | |
|---|---|
| Role model | Consciously practises nursing to a very high standard and conducts self in a way that the mentee can look to, value and adopt. |
| Energiser | Is enthusiastic about the whole of nursing, inspires interest and motivates mentee. |
| Envisioner | Is clear about how patient care could be even better, and is enthusiastic and dynamic about innovations. |
| Investor | Invests an appropriate amount of time in the mentee, and imparts own knowledge and experience. |
| Supporter | Encourages, gives time, is always willing to listen and makes himself or herself available in times of need. |
| Standard prodder | Always questioning standards of care and competence and is clear about own standards. |
| Teacher-coach | Teaches patient care-related knowledge and competence skilfully, gives guidance, allows time to practise and encourages the student to learn through experience. |
| Feedback giver | Provides positive feedback, points out weaknesses and discusses further learning. |
| Eye opener | Inspires interest in wider issues, political, financial, etc., and departmental initiatives that can impact on the clinical setting or specialism. |
| Door opener | Suggests available healthcare provisions and learning opportunities related to practice objectives. |
| Ideas bouncer | Encourages mentee to generate and verbalise new ideas, listens to them and helps mentee to reflect on them. |
| Problem solver | Helps the mentee to think systematically about problems and ways of resolving and preventing them. |
| Career counsellor | Available to offer own views and guidance in career planning |
| Challenger | Enables the mentee to think more critically about their decisions, and challenges views, opinions and beliefs. |

*Source:* Darling (1984).

*The mentor as the role model*

 **Think Point 1.1 – A role model**

Consider the terms *model* and *modelling*. Next consider what a role model is. Consider also why healthcare professionals need to be role models, who for, and what it is about a person that makes him or her a role model.

In response to Think Point 1.1, you might have felt that a mentor who is a role model is someone who fulfils NMC's (2006a) standards for mentors, as identified earlier in this chapter. Although the mentor would be a role model predominantly for clinical skills, they should also be a role model as an organizer of care, a researcher, and a teacher within the parameters of their post.

As with most nascent and tentative concepts, a concept analysis or a STEP (social, technical, economic and political) analysis can enable further clarification of the concept, a systematic understanding of various facets and components of the concept. Alternatively, a SWOT (strengths, weaknesses, opportunities and threats) analysis can be undertaken. Such an analysis can help the individual decide whether any problem-solving, avoidance or developmental actions need to be taken.

## Activity 1.4 – STEP analysis of role model

Using the headings social, technical, economic and political, conduct a STEP analysis of 'the mentor as a role model'.

Being a role model is a feature of Bandura's (1977) social learning theory, which stipulates that substantial learning occurs as a result of observation of appropriate professionals. Bahn (2001) suggests that role modelling is consistent with social learning theory, as substantial socialisation occurs in clinical learning environments. It is also a significant component of 'work-based learning', which is discussed in Chapter 4.

There can also be good role models, and bad role models, that is, how not to come over as a healthcare professional. Bad role models can therefore not be seen as a model at all, considering what the word 'model' means. A role model is 'an exemplary person or thing, a perfect exemplar of excellence' (Brown, 2002: 1806), that is, someone whose practice standards, attitudes and beliefs the observer can emulate. Individuals choose their role models, such as someone who is good at time management, at self-organisation, or in how they interact with colleagues.

Donaldson and Carter (2005) report on an evaluation of the perceptions of undergraduate students on role modelling within the clinical learning environment. They indicate that students stressed the importance of good role models whose competence they could observe and practise. Constructive feedback was needed on their practice from their role models to develop their competence and build their confidence, and to convert observed behaviour into their own behaviour and skill set.

Thomas (2005) reports that there are mixed views about nurses being role models of healthy habits when off duty. Faugier (2005a) suggests that role models are those whom we look up to, emulate and admire as professionals. However, in society in general, she suggests, people are basing their character identities, values and lifestyles

**Figure 1.3 Effects of support and challenge on the mentee's development**

*Source*: Daloz (1989).

on celebrities and characters in television programmes. This highlights how crucial the latter's public behaviours are. All teachers in the clinical setting (e.g. mentors) should therefore be aware of their impact as role models on students' learning of skills and professional attitudes.

*The mentor as a challenger and supporter*

---

### Think Point 1.2 – Mentoring support and challenge

Consider the characteristics of 'supporter' and 'challenger' identified by Darling (1984) and think of learning situations where you need to provide the mentee with a high level of challenge and support, and other situations where you afford low levels of each.

---

There are various examples of situations that present high or low challenge for learners in clinical settings, and the support required. Asking a third-year student nurse to consistently perform clinical skills for which they have already been signed as competent would provide a lesser challenge to them, and lesser support might be required. But if the same student hasn't yet learnt how to provide care in epidural pain control, for instance, then this would present a high challenge and the student is likely to need a high level of support. Daloz (1989) explored these two functions further and concluded that high support and challenge can lead to growth and achievement of vision, while low support and low challenge can result in stasis and apathy, as illustrated in Figure 1.3.

## Activity 1.5 – Ascertaining mentorship potential

Consider Darling's (1984) characteristics or roles of the mentor as detailed in Box 1.4, and identify situations where you needed to use these skills in relation to mentoring learners or of forthcoming opportunities for mentoring.

1. For each characteristic, do a self-rating of yourself as a mentor using numbers 1 to 4, 1 indicating development or learning need and 4 indicating skilled.
2. Next, focus on one or two of the skills on which you rate yourself as low, and consider why this is (e.g. lack of opportunity) and how you can develop this characteristic.

This exercise you have just undertaken is also referred to as 'measuring mentorship potential' (MMP) (Darling, 1984).

## Actions that support learning

## Activity 1.6 – Actions that support learning

Think of and make a list of a number of actions that can be taken by mentors that support learning.

No doubt a range of components that support learning can be identified. One of the key functions of the mentor is to help the student integrate into the practice setting, which entails managing the practice placement, receiving the student and conducting initial, mid-placement and final interviews, and possibly using learning contracts. Acceptance of the mentee (Rogers and Freiberg, 1994) signifies that the mentor accepts the student for their current levels of knowledge and competence, which may be extensive or minimal.

As for managing the placement, the designated mentor would have been nominated before the student starts on the placement and would need self-preparation time beforehand. Time would also have been set aside for receiving the student, and introducing them to the team, and associate mentors would have been identified.

Seeing the practice placement from a student's viewpoint suggests that they might be experiencing different feelings in anticipation of the placement. They are likely to appreciate any prior information sent to them, which might include any preparatory reading that the student can do. On the first day, they tend to appreciate an introduction to the clinical area, making them feel comfortable about learning, a friendly environment, student involvement, and continuity of mentorship. These perspectives are consistent with 'empathic understanding' identified as a key condition by Rogers and Freiberg (1994).

Furthermore, the NMC (2006a) indicates that to enable effective learning at least 40 per cent of the student's placement time must be spent working with the mentor. Similar rules apply to the practice teacher role. Previously the ENB (1997) had recommended that a mentor must work two shifts per week with the mentee. Moreover, the NMC (e.g. 2006a), and previously the Department of Health (1999), have identified the need for 'protected time' for mentoring. Mentoring can be made even more efficient by the use of learning contracts.

### Using learning contracts

Learning contracts are very much a feature of adult education (or andragogy – discussed in Chapter 2) and involve negotiated learning between teacher and student. As the word *contract* implies, a learning contract is a written and signed agreement between teacher (mentor in this case) and learner resulting in the latter's active involvement in decisions over practice objectives and other components of learning. Therefore it is often a feature of practice modules whereby the mentor and student agree on specific practice objectives and on the responsibilities of each party.

The use of learning contracts was advocated by Knowles et al. (1998) in the context of adult learners needing to exercise some self-direction in their learning. It constitutes an agreed set of objectives, which incorporates those of the course curriculum and those of the student, and formally recognises them. Therefore, the learning contract affords the student some control over their learning, stimulates their motivation to learn and to engage with the learning experience. It is also a medium for identifying the student's preferred learning style and, to some extent, the pace of their learning, and to explore the level of theory and practice integration.

However, the requirements and objectives set by the course curriculum have to be met. A learning contract section or pro forma may already have been included in the student's placement competencies booklet. Basically, the mentor and student discuss and agree what the student is aiming to learn, how the learning will take place, and how this will be evaluated. This is usually written down by the student and, when agreed, both mentor and student sign and date it. Learning pathways based on patient journeys can be incorporated as a strategy for achieving particular objectives. An example of a learning contract is presented in Box 1.5.

An alternative to a learning contract is a learning agreement (Open University, 2001; RCN, 2002), which has similar features but might not include signatures of those involved, nor rigid 'achieve-by' dates.

| Box 1.5 A learning contract | | | | |
|---|---|---|---|---|
| Name of student: | | | Cohort: | |
| Placement: | | | Mentor's name: | |
| Learning needs | Objectives | Resource and strategies | Target date | Evidence |
| What do I want to learn? – topic area | What do I want to have achieved at the end of my learning? – specific objectives | How will I learn, and who will help me? – learning strategies | Date of achieving learning | How will I know I have achieved my intended learning? |

Pre-contract

Signature of student:             Date:

Mentor's signature:             Date:

Name of link teacher/practice educator:      Name of personal tutor:

Comments on achievement of contract objectives

Signature of student:             Date:

Mentor's signature:             Date:

---

### Think Point 1.3 – The learning contract

What would logically happen after all three parties have signed the learning contract? Do you feel that it should be constantly reviewed to monitor the student's progress with its content, or only reviewed on the 'target date'?

---

Learning contracts may be seen by some as a chore. Others may prefer to write something treating it as a mere formality. But the benefits of learning contracts have been reported by Ghazi and Henshaw (1998), for instance, who found that learning contracts help to improve student attendance at lectures and student performance in assessments. Donaldson (1992), Northcott (1989) and others reported similar benefits.

An important step involved in constructing a learning contract is the mentor facilitating self-assessment by the student and identifying learning needs. Naturally, when a contract has been drawn up, then on the 'achieve-by' date there will be a need to ascertain whether the activities identified in the contract were undertaken and the objectives achieved. The review time will of course have been determined at the beginning when the content was being discussed and documented.

The mentor will have developed knowledge, understanding on use of learning contracts as part of the mentor preparation programme, along with how they can deliver these functions in the context of other roles that they have to fulfil.

Rogers and Frieberg (1994) indicate that learning contracts endow the student some freedom to learn aspects that they wish to learn and pursue areas that they find particularly interesting. A learning contract is also a medium for resolving any doubt that there may be about specific purposes of the learning experience. It clarifies the activities the student would engage in and provides motivation and reinforcement through the achievement of objectives.

Having determined that a contract can be a very useful educational tool, no doubt you'll be wondering what happens if the student does not take all the actions they had agreed to take or did not achieve all the specified objectives.

There are mixed views in the literature about whether learning contracts are legally binding. Mazhindu (1990) argues that they are, while Neary (2000a) suggests that this isn't the case. It is useful to note the NMC's (2005a) stance on record keeping, and the use of written records as evidence of actions taken or omitted. For learning contracts to be effective, they need to be skilfully constructed. Guidelines for constructing them are provided by Knowles (1990), Knowles et al. (1998) and the ENB (1987), and an example of a well-constructed learning contract is presented in Box 1.5.

## Adverse Effects of Poor Mentoring

A common experience in nursing in the twenty-first century is that nurses working in many clinical settings feel they are managing their workload with ongoing shortage of staff. Indeed Phillips et al. (2000) noted that mentors fulfil their mentoring role as one of several other roles they have during any span of duty. Despite 'protected time' for mentoring having been advocated for almost a decade (DoH, 1999; NMC, 2006a), the implementation of this remains very slow for many mentors due to the demands on their time. Knowingly or unknowingly, the mentor may be taking actions that discourage learning.

## Activity 1.7 – How the mentor might discourage learning

Think of, and make notes on, a range of actions on the part of mentors that, advertently or inadvertently, may be seen as discouraging or disabling learning.

The following case study presents an example of poor mentoring.

## Case Study – Poor mentoring

Mel Alexis is a second-year student nurse on a rehabilitation ward. One day she finished her shift early, having told the staff nurse in charge that she had a terrible headache, while in fact she was extremely upset regarding her placement.

That morning she had felt that the staff nurse had spoken to her in a very unprofessional manner, as she does to patients as well. This is what bothered Mel the most. She also challenged the staff nurse over her drug administration that morning. A patient was left her morning medication in a pot on the table, but was unable to swallow it as she needed assistance due to her having a weak side and problems with her other hand. As Mel walked past the patient's room, the patient called her and indicated that she had not taken her tablets yet. As Mel was not the nurse who administered the drugs, she called the nurse into the room for her to administer the drugs. The nurse said that she did not have time to do this but the tablets were correct for the patient. Mel agreed to assist in giving the medication but noticed three tablets lying on the table beside the pot. Mel asked the nurse what these tablets were and she advised they were morning medications as well. Mel doubted this as they were not in the medicine pot and asked the nurse why, but the latter did not give an answer and instead picked them up and put them into the pot. The nurse then told Mel to assist with the medications and Mel made it clear that she did not feel that the medications were correct, as there seemed to be more tablets than the patient usually took in the morning. The nurse told Mel not to question her drug administration so Mel felt she had no choice but to assist the patient in taking her drugs.

This event highlighted Mel's unhappiness with this ward. She had started feeling like this on day one when she was not introduced to any staff members or shown around. She had had to find things out for herself during her time on this ward and if she asked where something was, the staff said it would be quicker for them to get the item themselves rather than show Mel. As a second-year nurse, she was expecting to do many nursing activities but instead she felt she was treated like a support worker. Although Mel loves providing basic nursing care to patients, she expected a lot more out of this placement than she was actually achieving. Mel appreciates that on a rehabilitation ward nursing takes on a different role but she feels she has yet to see what this role is. Mel says she has always wanted to be a nurse and really loves the job, but this ward has now made her question this and it makes her very sad to feel like this.

There is a possibility that you have yourself witnessed poor mentoring, directly or indirectly. Other problems with mentoring remain prevalent. Earlier research into mentoring and assessing had identified personality characteristics that discourage learning. For instance, Darling's (1985) qualitative study revealed what she termed the characteristics of the 'galaxy of toxic mentors' (see Box 1.6).

---

### Box 1.6    The 'galaxy of toxic mentors'

| Types | Features |
|---|---|
| *Avoiders* | Mentors who are not available or accessible, also referred to as ignorers or non-responders. |
| *Dumpers* | Throw people into new roles or situations and let them flounder, either to sink or to swim, often deliberately. |
| *Blockers* | Actively avoid meeting the mentee's needs either by refusing requests, by controlling through withholding information, or by blocking the mentee's development by over-supervising. |
| *Destroyers/Criticisers* | Set out to destroy the mentee by subtle attacks to undermine confidence, and open and public verbal attacks and arguments, questioning of abilities and deliberately destroying confidence. |

---

In response to Activity 1.7, you may have felt that one of the problems that learners experience is the lack of opportunities to work with their named mentor. Other actions on the part of mentors that you might have thought of that can discourage learning are:

- lack of interest in students and in their learning needs;
- lack of knowledge about the student's course;
- lack of evidence-based practice or research utilisation;
- hierarchical and a lack of team approach;
- not acknowledging student's previous experience;
- negative attitudes;
- reluctant to change practice.

Based on extensive experience in management and the processes of decision making, Heirs and Farrell (1986) explored the mindsets of individual employees who enable an organisation to progress with its aims, and those of people who block this development. While the focus is on looking for and developing 'talents' in employees, the reality is that the mindset of some individuals can stifle development. These authors grouped the problematic or disabling traits, termed 'three mental poisons', as the functioning of rigid minds, ego minds, and Machiavellian minds (see Box 1.7). Such ways of thinking are not always obvious, nor easily detected, but do affect learning adversely.

---

### Box 1.7    The functioning of rigid minds, ego minds and Machiavellian minds

*The rigid mind:*

- Personal values are set or stereotyped
- Unable to see the positiveness in others' thoughts if they conflict with their thinking
- Continually blocks the openness of more creative thinking
- Loyal to traditional thinking and rejects novelty (seen as complexity)
- Appears to lack imagination or creativity
- Stifles use of originality and encourages complacency

*The ego mind:*

- Sees elements of a problem only in terms of self-interest and self-importance
- Fairly ambitious and has a reasonably high opinion of own abilities
- Looks after number one to the exclusion of other considerations
- Pays little attention to what others think and say
- Unsociable and does not contribute to collective thinking
- Will betray colleagues and even the organisation if it serves own ends

*The Machiavellian mind:*

- Quickly sees the range of likely outcomes of any decision
- Manipulates the feelings and ambitions of others to deceive
- Is devious and calculating
- Intimidates and engages in politicking
- Perpetuates worry in the organisations and is perpetually currying favour with superiors
- Scheming, cunning and suspicious of subordinates

*Source*: Heirs and Farrell (1986).

---

### Activity 1.8 – Mentors who disable learning

Discuss with a peer or in a small group why any mentor would behave in the negative ways described by Heirs and Farrell or Darling. Discuss if and how such behaviours can be changed.

Darling (1985) makes a number of suggestions on how to deal with toxic mentors. For instance, if the mentor–mentee allocation is unavoidable, then the mentee can try and keep the relationship balanced by building a support network with others, and drawing on own personal strengths. Heirs and Farrell (1986) suggest that it is the organisation's managers' responsibility to identify individuals who fall into any of these categories. Their 'poisonous' thinking endures, but can be changed gradually through formal and informal meetings. Decisions about delegation of responsibilities and roles need to be applied selectively.

## Approaches to Effective Mentoring

Despite the multiplicity of likely pitfalls that could inhibit learning, mentoring remains a necessary role for supporting learning in healthcare professions. A mentor in personal life is also advocated. Due to the humane, personal and suffering-prevention nature of healthcare provision, professional education programmes need to be appropriately structured and carefully monitored. Mentoring students must also be a structured or planned exercise, as discussed in this chapter. Furthermore, a small-scale study by van Eps et al. (2006) suggests that year-long mentorship programmes yield more beneficial outcomes for students in terms of the variety of skills that they acquired through the longer-term relationship than other ones.

However, the underlying principles on which each mentor bases their mentoring vary according to the personal beliefs and approaches of the mentor towards this role. The underpinning beliefs of the mentor about student learning therefore determine their approach to mentoring, and the model or framework of mentoring they use. The differences between the terms *approach*, *model* and *framework* are as follows. Approach to mentoring is personal to the mentor, and is based on his or her own life and professional experiences, personal views and beliefs. In mentoring, it would depend on the mentor's beliefs about nursing, pre-registration course design, student and learner populations and their styles of learning.

A model however is usually a research-deduced, and therefore informed, set of inter-related components that enable the activity to be addressed comprehensively. A framework takes this further, the components of the model being utilised as sections or headings for planning and implementing the activity, and may even have been empirically tested.

All three perspectives indicate a planned and systematic approach to the mentee's placement experience to make it more effective. Few frameworks for mentoring in healthcare are currently available. Darling's (1984) roles or characteristics of the mentor constitute such a model, the NMC's (2006a) standards for mentoring are another. Despite the pragmatic nature of frameworks, it is important to examine other approaches and models of mentoring that are available, such as those identified in Box 1.8.

---

### Box 1.8    Approaches, models and frameworks for mentoring

**Approaches to mentoring**

| | |
|---|---|
| *Classical mentoring* | Also known as informal or primary mentoring, is a natural, mutual and self-chosen relationship. |
| *Reflective mentoring* | Is based on learning theories, for example andragogy, styles of learning, and student-centred approaches; the mentor is a critical friend and co-enquirer. |

**Models or frameworks of mentoring**

| | |
|---|---|
| *Apprenticeship model* | The mentor is a skilled craftsperson, and the mentee learns by copying their actions. |
| *Competence-based model* | The mentor enables the mentee to achieve a set of practice objectives. |
| *Team-mentoring model* | A team of mentors mentors one or more students jointly, as recommended for nursing by, for example, Phillips et al. (2000) is akin to team supervision for doctorate students. |
| *Contract mentoring* | Formal mentoring that is time- or objectives-restricted, for example on placement at another institution. |
| *Pseudo-mentoring* | Also known as quasi or partial mentoring, in appearance only, and for a specific task such as dissertation supervision. |

---

A model is of course useful if it can be used as a framework for action. Kerry and Mayes (1995) tend to use the terms strategies, approaches and models interchangeably. They suggest four models of mentoring, namely the

- 'Colleagual model' – similar to team mentoring or the use of associate mentors.
- 'Counselling model' – refers to facilitation of learning using humanistic theories (discussed in Chapter 2).
- 'Professional model' – similar to the contract model, for example for a student on a practice placement, or in dissertation supervision (i.e. for a specific task).
- 'Process model' – also referring to facilitation of learning but enabling the mentee to eventually become an independent practitioner.

## Activity 1.9 – Application of models of mentoring

In your own experience of mentorship, which of these approaches, models or frameworks apply to learning professional skills in your own clinical setting, and why? Which ones suit you most? Make some notes.

It could be argued that often the apprenticeship model applies more to the training of support workers in that an apprentice normally learns skills and crafts at the level of task performance, along with associated practical knowledge, unlike the holistic psycho-bio-social approach taken by nurses. The competence model might apply to nursing but the reader needs to be aware of varying definitions of the term *competence*. Some definitions see competence as the ability to perform a skill in accordance with agreed procedures and incorporate practical knowledge, while others see it as including theoretical knowledge as well.

The reflective practitioner approach is one that is frequently favoured within health profession circles, and advocates the mentor taking a less directive approach to their practice-based teaching. Consider the following reflective recording in the portfolio of (Sheila) a student social worker'.

---

### Case Study – Sheila's portfolio

I visited Mr J while his care co-ordinator, who is also my practice supervisor, was on annual leave. At this time he expressed concern about his care co-ordinator and questioned her supportive abilities. My initial reaction was to explain that different practitioners would use different approaches, and advised him to raise the issue with the care co-ordinator. In a further conversation by telephone, Mr J reiterated the issue but in a more agitated manner and asked me to speak to the care co-ordinator. His care co-ordinator suggested that we visit Mr J to question him about what he actually wanted from the service and what type of support he felt she should offer. She felt Mr J didn't always engage with services (he frequently missed appointments), and that his drug addiction problem was the issue he most needed to address, but which she did not specialise in. Mr J was receiving services from the drug team but, again, he didn't always attend his appointments. However, it was clear Mr J felt he needed more support. As a result we discussed a referral to an agency which provided outreach support specifically for people with a history of offending and drug/alcohol abuse problems. Mr J was keen to accept this support

---

Reflective recordings provide an essential learning vehicle from clinical situations for mentees. The approaches and models presented in Box 1.8 may not all be seen as frameworks although they can be systematic and comprehensive. Most of the approaches are relatively recent concepts that await further empirical exploration or testing.

## Chapter Summary

This chapter has focused on mentoring as a concept and professional role. Having completed this chapter you will have learned about:

- The current and recent perspectives on the concept of mentoring, definitions of and distinctions between the mentor's and various related learning facilitation roles, such as assessors, preceptors, practice educators and supervisors, and those of the practice educator, link tutor and personal tutor. All these roles are established to facilitate healthcare learners learn clinical skills, knowledge and attitudes.
- A number of reasons why mentors are needed to support learners through preparatory healthcare programmes and practice placements, and the criteria for who can be a mentor.
- Effective mentoring, which encompasses effective working relationships, relevant mentor–mentee communication, and includes generic and specialist communication skills. The characteristics of mentors and enabling functions, which include the mentor as a role model for learners and ascertaining own mentorship potential. The actions that support learning including the use of learning contracts.
- Research findings on detrimental effects of poor, inefficient or adverse mentoring.
- The use of different models or approaches that identify mentors' perceptions of their mentoring role.

# TWO

# How Learners Learn

## Introduction

This chapter focuses on how healthcare professionals acquire the competence and knowledge required for patient or service user care delivery. It draws on multiple perceptions of learning, and covers:

- Precisely what healthcare learners learn in terms of different types of knowledge and professional skills, and what competence is.
- Different views and perspectives on what learning and education are and different learning strategies used by healthcare learners.
- Theories underpinning learning, in particular behaviourist, cognitive and humanistic learning theories, and their significance.
- How we learn healthcare skills, referring to major styles and approaches to learning, and how the mentor could adapt to students' styles and approaches.

As hands-on clinical intervention is the main part of healthcare professionals' jobs, an appropriate proportion of their preparatory courses is dedicated to this. In the nursing course, for instance, which amounts to a total of 4600 hours in three years, the NMC (2004b) requires half of this learning to be undertaken in the practice setting in direct patient care, and at least one-third on theoretical instruction. Learning in clinical settings therefore occupies a very significant role in pre-registration programmes. Consequently, this chapter and the next are based on the NMC's (2006a) competence criteria and outcomes under the domain 'facilitation of learning', which ecompasses:

1. *Competence*
   (a) Facilitate learning for a range of students, within a particular area of practice where appropriate, encouraging self-management of learning opportunities and providing support to maximise individual potential.

*Outcomes*
   (a) Use knowledge of the student's stage of learning to select appropriate learning opportunities to meet individual needs.

(b) Facilitate the selection of appropriate learning strategies to integrate learning from practice and academic experiences.

(c) Support students in critically reflecting upon their learning experiences in order to enhance future learning.

## Chapter outcomes

On completion of this chapter you should be able to:

1. Identify the specific knowledge and competence that healthcare profession learners obtain during their initial preparatory programmes.
2. Identify a range of meanings of the term *learning*.
3. Understand and analyse key theories of learning, and indicate how they can be applied to learning in clinical settings.
4. Comprehend the different styles and approaches to learning, and ways in which mentors can adapt their style of teaching to mentees' individual learning styles and approaches.

## What do Healthcare Learners Learn, and Why?

The first section of this chapter begins by identifying the specific knowledge and competencies that learners in healthcare professions learn, in particular during their initial preparatory programmes.

### Healthcare competencies

For nurse education programmes, the current pre-registration curriculum comprises four 'domains' of standards of proficiency (NMC, 2004b), which are:

1. professional and ethical practice;
2. care delivery;
3. care management;
4. personal and professional development.

Outcomes are identified under each of the four domains for the common foundation programme (CFP) (termed 'for entry to the branch programme') and for the four branches of mental health, adult, child and learning disabilities, for entry to the register. See Box 2.1 on p. 39 for standards for entry to the register for the adult branch, for instance.

The outcomes under each domain for the other branches, as well as for midwifery and SCPHNs, can be viewed in the relevant 'standards of proficiency' document which is available free from the NMC. 'Standards of Proficiency' for the preparation programmes of each AHP managed by the HPC have also been identified in appropriate HPC publications, namely those for (HPC, 2007):

- arts therapists;
- biomedical scientists;
- chiropodists/podiatrists;
- clinical scientists;
- dietitians;
- occupational therapists;
- operating department practitioners;
- orthoptists;
- paramedics;
- physiotherapists;
- prosthetists and orthotists;
- radiographers;
- speech and language therapists.

The General Medical Council and General Social Care Council publish similar standards. Other healthcare professionals such as clinical perfusion scientists, dance movement therapists, sports therapists, and complementary therapists, such as chiropractors, who normally already have their own separate professional body, can join the HPC at some point through a formal application and approval process. In addition to the regulatory bodies' standards, each healthcare profession's professional body, for example the Royal College of Nursing and the British Medical Association, tend to publish further guidance documents to enable implementation of the standards in professional preparation programmes.

## Why do people learn?

### Activity 2.1 – Reasons for learning

Take a step back and consider the learning we undertake in our professional lives, as well as in personal pursuits. Consider examples of what individuals learn, and why. Think of as many reasons as you can for individuals acquiring various forms of knowledge and skills, and make a list.

It could be argued that everyone learns throughout life – for example babies learn that, when they cry, this leads to food or comfort being made available to them. Younger adults learn new knowledge and skills to enable them, or to improve their chances of, gaining employment and thereby an income to be able to buy food and clothes for themselves, for instance. This could be seen as learning for self-preservation.

Another reason for learning could be self-betterment; self-actualisation is yet another. Professionals might learn more about their profession because they take pride in their craft, and want to acquire comprehensive relevant knowledge. Other reasons for professional and personal learning include:

- Curiosity – about particular subject areas.
- Need for more responsibility – for example through becoming a clinical manager.

**Box 2.1    Standards for entry to the adult branch of the register for the four domains**

1. **Professional and ethical practice**
   - Manage oneself, one's practice, and that of others, in accordance with the NMC's *Code of Professional Conduct*, recognising one's own abilities and limitations.
   - Practise in accordance with an ethical and legal framework which ensures the primacy of patient and service user interest and well-being and respects confidentiality.
   - Practise in a fair and anti-discriminatory way, acknowledging the differences in beliefs and cultural practices of individuals or groups.

2. **Care delivery**
   - Engage in, develop and disengage from therapeutic relationships through the use of appropriate communication and interpersonal skills.
   - Create and utilise opportunities to promote the health and well-being of patients, service users and groups.
   - Undertake and document a comprehensive, systematic and accurate nursing assessment of the physical, psychological, social and spiritual needs of patients, service users and communities.
   - Formulate and document a plan of nursing care, where possible in partnership with patients, service users, their carers and family and friends, within a framework of informed consent.
   - Based on the best available evidence, apply knowledge and an appropriate repertoire of skills indicative of safe nursing practice.
   - Provide a rationale for the nursing care delivered, which takes account of social, cultural, spiritual, legal, political and economic influences.
   - Evaluate and document the outcomes of nursing and other interventions.
   - Demonstrate sound clinical judgement across a range of differing professional and care delivery contexts.

3. **Care management**
   - Contribute to public protection by creating and maintaining a safe environment of care through the use of quality assurance and risk-management strategies.
   - Demonstrate knowledge of effective inter-professional working practices which respect and utilise the contributions of members of the health and social care team.
   - Delegate duties to others, as appropriate, ensuring that they are supervised and monitored.
   - Demonstrate key skills.

4. **Personal and professional development**
   - Demonstrate a commitment to the need for continuing professional development and personal supervision activities in order to enhance knowledge, skills, values and attitudes needed for safe and effective nursing practice.
   - Enhance the professional development and safe practice of others through peer support, leadership, supervision and teaching.

- Saving time and effort – students can gain a great deal of knowledge and understanding in one lecture, which would take them a very long time to acquire by self-study.
- Enhancing one's skills – to become even more competent, and even an expert.
- Sense of achievement – by having developed new skills, for instance.
- Acquisition of new skills – in chosen areas of interest.

## The student's learning needs: knowledge and competence

In addition to the placement competencies that students are required to learn, they are likely to have their own aims and thoughts on specific healthcare knowledge and competence that they'd wish to acquire during particular clinical placements, especially as adult learners (Knowles et al., 1998). This should be encouraged and opportunities for learning identified, as appropriate.

Students acquire knowledge in, say, human physiology, pharmacology and treatment methods, that is consistent with the outcomes under the four domains identified by the NMC (2004b). The terms *competency* and *competency* are often used in relation to the skills they develop. Types of knowledge are discussed shortly, but first what do the terms competence and competency mean?

### Defining competence
There are conflicting definitions of the terms competence and competency in the literature.

---

### ⸛⃰ Think Point 2.1 – Being competent

Focusing on your own experience of working with colleagues in your healthcare profession, and of students approaching the end of their courses, consider what being competent means. For example, which pay band, or what amount of experience makes a healthcare professional 'competent'?

---

Although the term *competence* is used rather glibly, it is a term that has several definitions, as identified by Bradshaw (1997), for instance. Benner (2001) sees being competent as being at the midway point in the stages of skill acquisition. This is the point when the learner is deemed able to perform the skill unsupervised, but further learning is required to become 'proficient' or 'expert'.

Benner (2001) suggests that competence is an interpretively defined area of skilled performance identified and described by its intent, function and meanings (as in competency statement). Policy and research documents therefore indicate that the terms *competence* and *competent* apply to the person, that is, the professional's overall knowledge, skills and attitudes, and their 'fitness to practise'. The term *competency*, on the other hand, applies to specific clinical skills, which in nursing also include the associated knowledge and attitude components.

The NMC (2005b) identifies competence as relating to the student demonstrating their 'capability' in certain skill areas to a required standard at a particular point in time, and that competencies are component skills that contribute to being competent and to achieving the standards of proficiency for registration. A widely accepted definition of competence is 'a term used to describe the skills and ability to practise safely and effectively without the need for direct supervision' (UKCC, 1999: 35). The concept of competence is fundamental to the autonomy and accountability of healthcare professionals, and therefore to their codes of conduct or practice (e.g. NMC, 2007).

The NMC (2004c) sees a competent nurse as one who consistently demonstrates fitness for practice. Essentially, it can be argued that competence implies being able to perform the skill according to the approved procedure and without the need for direct supervision. Others argue that competence refers to the ability or capability and the associated practical knowledge, and yet others feel that competence signifies having theoretical knowledge as well. As a term that is also used in NVQ and in medical education, its profession-specific definition should be accepted, in that in the former the remit for NVQ courses signifies the ability to perform the relevant skill and having the associated practical knowledge. In medical and non-medical professions, competence signifies having the ability, the practical and theoretical knowledge.

On the other hand, 'lack of competence' is seen as 'a lack of knowledge, skill or judgement of such a nature that the registrant is unfit to practise safely and effectively in any field in which the registrant claims to be qualified, or seeks practise' (NMC, 2004c: 3). Peers, managers and employers as well as the general public are expected to report lack of competence through the appropriate channels.

### Types of knowledge associated with professional skills

The knowledge required for clinical competence can be grouped or classified in different ways. Schon (1995) notes that healthcare professionals have an accumulated repertoire of knowledge, with mastery over its manipulation, production and application. Benner (2001) identifies practical knowledge and theoretical knowledge, as well as tacit knowledge. She suggests that novices, that is, healthcare professionals who are new to healthcare, are more inclined to use rules and guidelines, such as practical knowledge, while 'expert' healthcare practitioners tend to use intuition more.

Different types of knowledge base that professionals use can also be viewed from Carper's (1978) 'patterns of knowing' perspective. They are:

- *Empirical knowledge:* knowledge derived from research and scientific experiments, which therefore can be measured, tested and corroborated.
- *Ethical knowledge:* knowledge based on morals and philosophy, but which is usually difficult to test.
- *Aesthetic knowledge:* knowledge based on sensitivity or intuition, also referred to as the 'art of nursing'.
- *Personal knowledge:* knowledge of one's self and how it influences one's professional practice.

Each of these 'patterns' is seen as equally important for healthcare practice and for developing further knowledge. Therefore in relation to physiotherapy and knowledge regarding hip replacement, for instance, empirical knowledge relates to the research evidence for hip replacement operations, the patient experiencing less chronic pain and a better quality of life afterwards. Ethical knowledge could refer to whether, say, an 80-year-old widow consents to such an operation, and whether it is right to subject her to such a potentially traumatic experience. Aesthetic knowledge refers to the expertise and extensive experience of the physiotherapist to enable the patient to mobilize fully after the operation. Personal knowledge refers to the physiotherapist knowing himself or herself as a person, their preferences, values and the effect these might have on their professional practice.

The mentor's role towards the physiotherapy student would be to enable the mentee to acquire skills and practical knowledge, but includes having a good insight into the mentee's level of scientific, ethical, and personal knowledge.

Alternatively, Scheler (1980) classified knowledge according to the rate at which it alters, that is, according to their 'artificiality'. Technological knowledge such as knowledge of medical devices is seen as the most artificial, as they change frequently through new inventions; and knowledge of human anatomy for instance is more enduring.

In a study exploring whether nurses use knowledge from research findings to inform decision making, Thompson et al. (2002) found that although colleagues are the more immediate source of information on which to base decisions, they are also a source of research (or data-based empirical) knowledge and useful networks. However, although various decisions made by clinical managers are based on empirical knowledge, other decisions are influenced by experience and intuition.

## Major Views and Perspectives on Learning, Teaching and Education

### What is learning?

How individuals learn has been researched and defined over a number of years. So what is learning? How do you define 'learning'? Generally dictionaries provide a broad explanation of the term. For instance, to learn is to 'acquire knowledge (of a subject) or skill as a result of study, experience or instruction; to acquire or develop the ability to do' (Brown, 2002: 1562). More specific definitions have come from philosophers and educational psychologists. The latter generally agree that learning is a process which leads to modification in behaviour or the acquisition of new abilities or responses, and which is additional to natural development, growth or maturation.

Accordingly Gagné (1983) defined learning as a change in human disposition or capability, which persists over a period of time and which is not simply ascribable to the process of growth. Curzon (2001: 11) defines learning as 'the apparent modification of a person's behaviour through his activities and experiences, so that his knowledge, skills and attitudes, including modes of adjustment, towards his environment are changed, more or less permanently'.

These definitions tend to concur that:

- learning is reflected in changes in behaviour, physical and attitudinal;
- learning occurs in day-to-day life experiences, in addition to planned formal education;
- learning a psychomotor skill is permanent in nature in that the individual subsequently has the capacity to perform the skilled act at a future point in time.

Specialist skills may 'decay' mainly due to environmental factors such as changes in medical devices, social values and so on. Learning in healthcare professions is about learning competence and knowledge, the nature of which was discussed earlier. In healthcare professions, learning is a lifelong process of skill and knowledge acquisition and updating them through planned participation in focused reading and structured programmes of study.

## Perspectives on learning

Learning experiences are influenced by where the learner 'is coming from', as each person perceives new experiences in a different way, depending on how they relate to their past. However, two opposing views about learning are suggested by Ramsden (1988), who identifies learning as either (a) a quantitative accretion of facts and procedures, or (b) a change in the way in which people understand the world around them.

Education, on the other hand, according to Socrates (2000 years ago), is not merely transferring knowledge of facts and procedures from 'teacher' to 'pupil'. Rather it is 'an adventure, an activity of the mind, a pursuit demanding reflection, analysis and investigation, a social activity undertaken by equals freely associated to engage in dialogue' (Jeffs, 2003: 28).

Radical distinctions were also made by Freire (1996), who argued that there were two contrasting perspectives on education and learning, which he identified as the 'banking' concept of education versus 'problem posing'. The banking concept, as the traditional mode of learning, involves the teacher helping a student fill their minds with knowledge, which is later '*cashed out*' relatively unchanged, for example in examinations. The problem-posing approach to education, on the other hand, is education through dialogue. Facilitator and students meet and exchange ideas and experiences through critical discussions and debate. Neither facilitator nor student necessarily has the 'right' answer as there is room for 'multiple realities'.

Another perspective is provided by Peters (1966, 1973) regarding the differentiation between training and education. What distinctions would you draw between education and training? Peters (1966) notes that training means knowledge and skill devised to bring about some specific end. The aims of education on the other hand, he notes, are that:

- something of value is being passed on and learned;
- the individual comes to care about the learning involved, to develop understanding, and to achieve;
- what is being learned must have a place in a coherent pattern of life, that is, relevance among other things in life.

Therefore, education 'implies that something worthwhile is being, or has been, intentionally transmitted in a morally acceptable manner ... The educated person is one whose life has been transformed by the deepening and widening of his understanding and sensitivity. To be educated is not to arrive at a destination; it is to travel with a different view' (Peters, 1973: 122).

These perspectives on learning correspond with the concepts of teacher-centred learning and student-centred learning, which are discussed in Chapter 3. So how do the definitions and these views on learning and education apply to or compare with approaches taken in healthcare profession education curricula?

### Activity 2.2 – Different perspectives on nurse education

Discuss with a course or work-based peer your thoughts on how far Ramsden's (1988), Freire's (1996) and Peters's (1966, 1973) perspectives on learning apply to nursing, midwifery or an AHP education.

In nurse education, the difference between education and training is that the word 'training' is usually associated with a well-defined course of action with a definite end point, which is usually that of developing certain pre-defined skills (Burnard and Chapman, 1990). It is said to be a convergent process in that everyone undertaking the training ends up with mostly the same skills and abilities and the same ways of performing them. Education, on the other hand, is a divergent process of developing and deepening knowledge, skills, interests and values, for instance. Education does not stop at a pre-determined point of attainment, but more in the development of critical ability and, consequently, the individual remains open to new impressions, principles and perspectives. Education facilitators should therefore provide an environment where students feel supported sufficiently to decide on areas of learning, as long as the core curriculum aims are achieved.

## Where do healthcare learners learn?

Naturally, learning doesn't occur only in university classrooms through lectures, workshops and books, but it also occurs in work-based settings, during patient or service user contact. Learning also occurs in skill laboratories and in the ward teaching room or office. Furthermore, learning occurs in the trust's post-graduate or in-service training departments. In the clinical setting, learning can take the form of informal and structured teaching sessions.

Furthermore, learning occurs in the student common room, in informal social meetings and even 'in car parks, in corridors, over tea as well as through unnoticed patterns of behaviour and interaction in the classroom itself' (Field, 1999: 12). This notion that learning can occur from friends and peers, and in a whole gamut of settings is referred to as social capital (Gopee, 2002a). A corresponding notion is human capital, which refers to self-investment of time and effort by individuals through learning in university or public libraries, as well as at home, and the non-traditional places suggested by Field (1999). Learning occurs everywhere, including in therapeutics, propaganda practices, for example. Learning contributes to progress, and notions such as learning society and learning organisation (most companies have training and customer services departments) have evolved.

## Theories Underpinning Learning

There are a number of theories of learning that can underpin professional education programmes. Exploration of these theories has taken place over several decades. It has swung between theories of learning, models of learning, principles of learning and styles of learning, with theories and styles of learning being the more popular concepts in the twenty-first century. Further concepts related to learning theories are:

- *Situated learning* – learning in social groups, communal knowledge, apprenticeship.
- *Tacit learning* – knowledge that is implicit and not easily explained.
- *Existential learning* – learning from being and deriving meaning from it.
- *Psychoanalytic learning* – conscious–unconscious dynamics are explored, resulting in a more integrated person.
- *Trait modification* – developing personality characteristics.

Situated learning approach, for instance, comprises learning sub-concepts in social groups or settings, and includes communal knowledge and apprenticeship (Burgoyne and Reynolds, 1997), learning about the ways of the subculture, for example in a small community hospital. Other concepts related to learning are: andragogy, student-centred and teacher-centred education, objectives and learning outcomes, taxonomy levels, reflective learning, practice-focused and work-based learning, evidence-based learning, motivation theories and learning by trial and error. Most of these are referred to at appropriate points in the book.

There are at least ten schools of thought, theories or models of learning. They have all created different definitions, and incorporate some of the concepts identified earlier. The more robust learning theories are:

- behaviourist learning theories;
- cognitive learning theories;
- humanistic learning theories.

### Behaviourist learning theories

Most learning theories belong to the field of psychology, which in the earlier part of the twentieth century used to be about introspection, that is, how mental processes are structured. However, gradually there was a move away from this paradigm (e.g. Watson, 1978) and it was suggested that psychology should be a science, and psychological theories should be based on observable and quantifiable data, that is, those manifested in changes in behaviour. Initially psychologists worked with animals to observe behaviour changes, and later with people.

Behaviourist learning theories refer to learning through response to particular stimuli, resulting in classical conditioning or operant conditioning. Classical conditioning refers to change in behaviour through stimulus–response, whereby desirable responses to particular stimuli, that is, newly learned behaviours are rewarded. Operant conditioning is a subsequent development by Skinner (1971) and others, whereby approximations of desired behaviour are rewarded, and thereby the target behaviour develops gradually. Being rewarded for new learning is also known as positive reinforcement, and can be external, in the form of verbal affirmations from the teacher (or close relatives) such as 'well done', or material rewards, or they can be internal through self-satisfaction.

Behaviourist learning theory can be applied to healthcare professionals' education programmes. For instance, operant conditioning can be effectively applied when students with weak academic backgrounds could achieve high levels in academia if earlier attempts are positively reinforced. Overall, healthcare learners are positively reinforced both by feeling a sense of achievement on being able to perform new healthcare skills, and by their mentors/supervisors acknowledging or recognising their newly developed competence.

Another example is that gaining praise for becoming competent at a particular clinical skill, or part-skills towards the desired competent performance, can positively motivate the student and make them want to learn new skills. Thus praiseworthy performance or approximations of competent practice or of part-skills by healthcare learners are rewarded or positively reinforced.

Social learning theory builds on these early behaviourist theories whereby the individual observes competent behaviour or skill performance by professionals, learns and reproduces it, and if the attempt is positively reinforced then that behaviour or skill is likely to be adopted. It refers to behaviour, attitudes and values of teachers or other role models that may be copied by learners (Bandura, 1977, 1986) and thus learned in social situations, as discussed in Chapter 1.

## Cognitive learning theories

As just indicated, behaviourist learning theories initially constituted an attempt to make psychology more scientific and empirical. More recently, various education sectors, including nurse education, have incorporated aspects of behaviourist theories and social learning theory into professional education programmes.

Subsequent work by Piaget (1962), Ausubel et al. (1978) and others led to the evolution of cognitive learning theories, which takes the view that learning is an internal purposive action involving thinking, perception, information processing and memory. Cognitive learning theories include:

- Gestalt theory of learning – entailing insightful learning, the 'aha' phenomenon.
- Ausubel et al.'s (1978) assimilation theory – which incorporates information processing.
- Experiential learning – learning through engaging in practical activities, followed by reflection.

Cognitive learning theories were initially based on animal experiments by Kohler (1925), but all three theories can be applied to healthcare professional education programmes. They include learning by insight (or insightful learning). Gestalt learning theory refers to seeing the whole picture, and insight is gained through the 'aha' phenomenon and the sudden realisation of a solution to a problem, for instance the 'penny-dropping' experience.

Gestalt theory of learning can be applied to professional education programmes by structuring learning so that learners are given problem situations to resolve; through group discussions and a process of insightful learning, and experiencing the 'aha' phenomenon, learning can occur. Group discussions, project work, self-directed learning and peer learning can enable this process. This can be used in teaching, for instance by asking a small group of students to resolve a snapshot of a clinical situation such as helping a patient with partial paralysis move from a bed to a chair.

To a good extent, Bruner's (1960) discovery learning theory refers to insightful learning. It involves situations that are devised in such a way that the learner can discover principles and underlying techniques for themselves. It also involves the use of past experience and existing knowledge to form new insights. For instance, a student who witnesses a patient with asthma gain relief from distressed breathing by using their inhaler can gain further insight into the specific functions of bronchioles and alveoli in oxygen transfer previously encountered in books or lectures.

Ausubel et al.'s (1978) assimilation theory is based on the view that most meaningful cognitive learning takes place as a result of interaction between the knowledge (cognitive structures) the individual already possesses, and new information that the individual encounters. Thus the single most important factor influencing learning is what the learner already knows. This forms the basis for the transfer of learning, in that, for instance, once the learner comprehends the principles of asepsis in hospital settings the knowledge can be adapted in community settings.

Ausubel et al.'s (1978) assimilation theory refers to activating the relevant knowledge the student already has so as to assimilate new knowledge into their existing mental structures. This also increases retention. It is also relevant for adult learners, as they already have substantial knowledge prior to starting on an academic course.

For new information to be 'received and assimilated', or subsumed into an anchoring structure, or schema, Ausubel and colleagues suggest giving the learner prior reading or the opportunity to engage in particular activities in preparation for the teaching session (referred to as 'advanced organisers'). The advanced organiser creates an anchoring structure for the new knowledge, like a scaffolding of ideas on which to build what the student needs to know. For instance, prior to a practice placement with a physiotherapist, the learner could be advised to revise or learn about the microstructure of muscles, in readiness for learning how they are strengthened through exercises by a patient who has suffered a fracture of the shin bone.

Cognitive learning theory therefore involves learning by participation and continually taking into consideration the person's previous knowledge and competence, such as clinical skills already learnt by the student on previous placements, and university skills' laboratories.

Experiential learning refers to learning by doing, rather than by merely being informed by others about a particular topic. It is achieved by building simulation activities in teaching–learning sessions, for instance, as advocated by Kolb (1984) among others. Experiential learning is therefore a component of reflective learning.

**Think Point 2.2 – Learning from experience**

Consider the question 'Do we learn from all experiences we come across in our day-to-day activities?'

In his study of experiences that individuals encounter as they go about their normal day-to-day business, and how much they learn from them, Jarvis (1995) deduced a typology of learning, which identifies three categories and nine types of potential learning experiences (see Box 2.2.)

---

Box 2.2   A 'typology of learning'

| Category of response | Type of learning/non-learning |
| --- | --- |
| *Non-learning* | Presumption |
| | Non-consideration |
| | Rejection |
| *Non-reflective learning* | Pre-conscious learning |
| | Skills learning |
| | Memorisation |
| *Reflective learning* | Contemplation |
| | Reflective skills learning |
| | Experimental learning |

*Source:* Jarvis (1995).

---

The typology also acknowledges the reality that there are particular situations that do not lend themselves to much learning for particular individuals, that is, non-learning experiences. The second category in the typology is non-reflective learning, which includes rote learning and memorising, for example temporary or one-off use of telephone numbers.

However, the third category is reflective learning, which focuses on the important part that experience plays in the learning process. Kolb (1984), for instance, suggests that learning can be conceived as a four-stage learning cycle (see Figure 2.1) that involves identifying the immediate concrete experience as the basis for observation and reflection. Out of this arise new concepts for hypothesis and theory building. Implications of these are considered in new situations and then theory is confirmed, adjusted or advanced.

This form of learning is widely used in general and professional education programmes. Individuals are encouraged to learn from situations or 'critical incidents' they encounter, to analyse them in the context of published literature, and to record

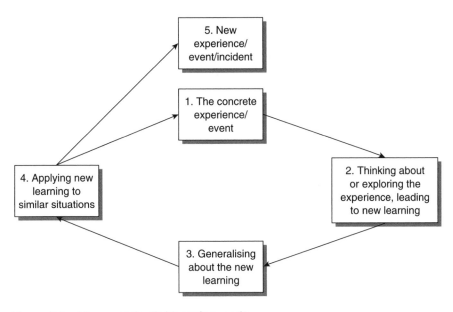

**Figure 2.1   The experiential learning cycle**

*Source*: adapted from Kolb (1984).

them systematically in their portfolios. These can comprise assessed work components of their programme of study.

The rationale for reflective practice in healthcare is that it is a means of constructing or generating knowledge from particular incidents. The origins of reflection on incidents go back to times when, for instance, techniques for dealing with aggressive behaviour in mental health nursing were minimal. When clinical staff met after such incidents to discuss the situation, they started to realize that if cues and signs of potential violence were identified in the individual patient before the disruptive incident actually occurred, then they could take certain actions to prevent it happening in the first place. This was formalized and seen as a therapeutic means that could be used step by step to prevent the disruptive incident. This also constituted constructing knowledge from clinical practice. The lack of knowledge and theory development from day-to-day experiences in clinical setting was a weakness identified by Phillips et al.'s (2000) study of mentoring practices.

Similar 'concrete experiences' led to changes in clinical practice such as use of triage system in Accident and Emergency departments, ensuring normal saline solution is at room temperature or above, prior to using it for wound cleansing. Several of these examples are noted in Chapter 5.

Kolb's (1984) learning cycle comprises four stages in the learning process, from the initial concrete experience or event to applying new learning to similar new situations. A fifth step can be added to this learning cycle to signify that if learning from the reflection does not seem to apply to another similar situation, then the latter becomes a new critical incident to learn from.

Teachers and students can utilise the model of reflection adapted by Boud et al. (1985), Gibbs (1988), or others that are generally available in the literature. Boud and colleagues' model of reflective practice involves identifying the concrete experience, observation and reflections, attending to feelings, re-evaluating the experience, and new learning.

For instance, when the student encounters a new experience during the clinical placement, they observe the experience as a critical incident and later they recall the incident, and describe it, reflect on it and explore it in the context of existing knowledge within professional and relevant literature. As a result of this, they develop and generate further insight by identifying and redefining the problem in a climate of mutual support (at university reflection-on-action workshops, for instance). They can share their new-found knowledge in as much detail as appropriate, even make a presentation, as it might have teaching implications for future practice. However, to benefit from this concept, the scheduling of the learning process should ensure that time is made available following clinical placements for reflection, consolidation and evaluation.

## Humanistic learning theories

A third group of theories that have been developed about how learning occurs is humanistic learning theories, which include:

- Alan Rogers's characteristics of adult education and andragogy;
- Carl Rogers's student-centred approach to learning;
- Maslow's learning as self-actualisation.

Humanistic learning theorists claim that preceding theories omit aspects of human existence such as feelings, attitudes and values, and thereby overlook the more holistic perspective that incorporates attitudinal components of learning. They suggest that learning should be concerned with personal human growth. Students learn concepts, theories, models and propositions (i.e. 'propositional knowledge') from books and other learning resources, and spend more classroom time on experiential learning activities, which include thinking processes that also incorporate exploration of values, attitudes and feelings.

### Adult education
In the context of the more holistic and humanistic approaches to learning, adult learning is another concept in its own right.

---

 **Think Point 2.3 – Adult learners**

Consider the question 'Should ways of teaching adults be different from ways of teaching school children or college students?' That is, what is different about adult students in contrast to school or college pupils? Think of reasons for your answer.

**Table 2.1   Differences between how adults and children learn**

| How children learn | How adults learn |
| --- | --- |
| • Children have shorter attention spans, and therefore a variety of learning activities is needed, including starter activities<br>• Teaching children is pedagogy, e.g. telling them<br>• Children are more open to new ideas<br>• There is a need to reinforce information over time | • Adults are (usually) self-motivated to learn<br>• Adults may have relevant professional and life experiences<br>• Open discussion is more feasible in adult groups<br>• Lesson content can be adjusted based on ongoing evaluation of learning needs |

Rogers (2002), Mezirow (1983) and Knowles et al. (1998) suggest various ways in which teaching adults, or adult education, is different from teaching children. Teaching adults includes teaching university students on generic or professional courses. Some of the differences suggested by nurses on post-registration courses are identified in Table 2.1.

However, in both instances, the learner–teacher relationship is important and needs to be based on mutual trust. Different teachers may have their own repertoire of different teaching styles and techniques when teaching adult students. Rogers's (2002) research concludes by identifying the characteristics of adult students or learners, as:

- Individuals define themselves, and have a self-image as adult students.
- They are in the middle of a process of growth, not at the start of the process.
- They bring with them a package of experience and values.
- They come to learning with intentions.
- Learners bring with them expectations about the learning process.
- Learners have competing interests.
- Learners already have their own set of patterns of learning.

Adult education is defined by Mezirow (1981) as an organised and sustained effort to assist adults to learn in a way that enhances their capacity to function as self-directed learners. Both Mezirow's definition and Rogers's characteristics of adult learners suggest that adult students' learning can be facilitated more effectively within an ethos of self-directed learning. Mentors can build self-directed learning into practice placement programmes for learners by allocating time for exploring further relevant clinical experiences or consulting relevant learning resources.

 **Think Point 2.4 – Adult education in healthcare courses**

How far is the adult learning approach relevant or applicable to nursing and other AHP education?

*Andragogy and self-directed learning*

Andragogy is an approach to teaching and learning aimed at enabling individuals to become aware that they should be the originators of their own thinking. Accordingly, although substantial knowledge and skill acquisition begins on qualifying (or becoming a registered nurse), it is up to the individual professional to determine the necessary areas of learning for themselves. This learning could be instigated by ward-based experiences, and the self-direction developed should become career-long.

A qualitative study of lecturers' and students' perceptions of self-directed learning and factors that facilitate or impede them, by Lunyk-Child et al. (2001), revealed that students who engage in self-directed learning undergo a transformation that begins with negative feelings (i.e. confusion, frustration and dissatisfaction) but ends with confidence and skills for lifelong learning.

However, another side to self-directed learning is highlighted by Hughes (1999) who indicates that this approach is not necessarily 'emancipatory', as it can be a 'repressive instrument' in that it can marginalise the significance of collective and co-operative learning, that is, learning in groups. Hughes suggests that governments can use self-directed learning to argue that less central funding would be required to educate self-directed learners. Furthermore, Knowles et al. (1998) suggest that the teacher needs to develop specific competencies to implement self-directed learning effectively. In the light of these issues and reservations related to andragogy, and the benefits, it can be concluded that in healthcare:

- Adult education constitutes collaborative activities by teachers and learners.
- Teaching should build on learners' professional experiences.
- Learners should participate in identifying learning needs, setting objectives and evaluating learning.
- The level of effective application of theory to clinical practice must always be identified.
- The role of the teacher is that of a facilitator.
- The outcome of the teaching and learning encounter should be to enable the individual to develop into a responsible autonomous practitioner.

## Student-centred approach to learning

Carl Rogers (1983) is well known for suggesting that teaching may be an overrated activity, as it is learning that should be in focus. For this to happen, he advocated the use of empathic understanding, genuineness, and being non-judgemental in learning situations. These activities are helping skills that Rogers successfully transferred from therapeutic counselling situations to student learning situations (Rogers and Freiberg, 1994). The teacher thus becomes the facilitator of student-centred learning, as is also advocated by Knowles et al. (1998) and Freire (1996). The facilitator achieves this by creating the environment for learning, and empowering students to become responsible, to develop self-awareness and to think of alternatives. Student-centred teaching is discussed in some detail in Chapter 3.

*Learning and self-actualisation*

Maslow's (1987) theory of a hierarchy of human needs suggests that our highest-level need, which is also lower priority, is our need for self-actualisation. Our physiological needs are highest priority, followed by safety needs, the need for belongingness and love, our self-esteem needs, and finally the need for self-actualisation. It could be argued that the goal of education is to assist individuals to achieve self-actualisation, to help the person to become the best that they are able to become. Maslow observed that the characteristics of self-actualising individuals are that they:

- have a more efficient perception of reality;
- demonstrate acceptance of self and others;
- show spontaneity, simplicity and naturalness;
- are problem-centred;
- possess a quality of detachment and have a need for privacy;
- exercise autonomy, independence of culture and environment;
- show continued freshness of appreciation;
- have peak experiences;
- experience deeper, more profound interpersonal relations;
- demonstrate democratic character;
- have a philosophical, non-hostile sense of humour;
- show creativeness;
- seem to transcend any culture.

Teachers might argue that they apply the already discussed learning theories as appropriate with particular groups or with individual learners. However, from adult educators' professional perspectives, andragogy also requires consideration of whether the adult student is merely biologically adult, or merely of legally adult age, or is also being a psychologically and socially responsible adult.

## How Else do We Learn Healthcare Skills?

In addition to different theories of how learning occurs, there are also different styles and approaches to learning adopted by individuals. The distinctions between theories and styles can be explained as follows.

A theory tends to imply cause and effect, that is, if we do x, then y will happen. For instance, if the Smiths send their child to an independent school, then he/she will have a better chance of securing a student place in a reputable university. According to the dictionary (Brown, 2002: 3236) a theory is 'a systematic statement of rules or principles to be followed; a system of ideas or statement explaining something, especially one based on general principles independent of the thing to be explained'. Alternatively, Lindberg et al. (1998: 62) define a theory as 'a group of concepts, definitions, and statements that presents an organised view of phenomena ... with the intent of describing, explaining, or controlling these phenomena'. A learning theory, the humanistic theory for instance, comprises an organised view of a group of concepts that should result in much more effective learning.

In contrast to a learning theory, a learning style refers to the unique way in which the particular individual tends to respond to learning situations. For instance, do they accept new learning instantly or do they prefer to reflect on it first? Do they question first whether the learning has practical applications or do they accept new concepts at theoretical levels? Alternatively, approaches to learning tend to depend on the level of individual commitment to particular episodes of learning.

## Major learning styles

> **Think Point 2.5 – How do you prefer to learn? What is your learning style?**
>
> We are all unique as learners. How do each of us prefer to learn? What is your preferred learning style? Which style does not suit you?

Learning styles have been researched over a number of years, and Honey and Mumford's (2000) classification of styles of learning is one that has been most widely published. You might have responded to Think Point 2.5 by identifying that you prefer to learn by attending a course or lecture, that is, in formal teaching situations. Others may prefer to learn by:

- watching others first;
- trial and error, generally through experience;
- reading and other forms of personal study such as distance learning;
- discussion with others.

Another well accepted proponent of learning styles is Kolb (1984), whose theory of learning and identification of learning styles is based on a view of learning as a series of experiences with cognitive additions to existing psychological structures. There are some similarities in the way Kolb and then Honey and Mumford group different learning styles. Kolb suggests that there are four styles of learning manifested by students, namely the converger, the diverger, the assimilator and the accommodator. Honey and Mumford (2000) suggest that individual learners vary between whether they are activists, reflectors, theorists or pragmatists. Jarvis and Gibson (1997) add other learning styles such as focusers, scanners, impulsivity and reflectivity. The main learning styles are summarised in Box 2.3.

---

**Box 2.3   Major learning styles**

*Converger vs Diverger*   Convergers are individuals who tend to use abstract thinking, progress to active experimentation, and generate a single correct solution; divergers tend to start from concrete experiences, generate ideas, then speculate on broader perspectives.

*(Continued)*

| | |
|---|---|
| *Impulsivity vs Reflectivity (similar to Accommodator vs Assimilator)* | Using the 'impulsive' style means the individual tends to respond first, at times spontaneously, and reflect later; those who use reflectivity tend to reflect first and respond subsequently. |
| *Activists vs Reflectors* | Individuals who are activists tend to fully involve themselves in new experiences; reflectors ponder on experiences from different perspectives, thoroughly collecting and analysing them, and identifying further learning from them. |
| *Theorists vs Pragmatists* | Theorists are individuals who start from observations, and develop or synthesise them into theories; pragmatists tend to consider new ideas and techniques in the context of their application to practice situations. |
| *Focuser vs Scanner* | Focusers are individuals who examine the whole problem and develop solutions from them; scanners tend to solve one aspect of the problem at a time and assume it is the correct one unless it is disproved. |
| *Holistic vs Serialistic* | Individuals using the holistic approach tend to prefer to see a phenomenon as a whole, while serialists prefer to identify its components and their roles as part of the whole phenomenon. |

Styles of learning are explained in full detail in relevant literature. For instance, the style *Impulsivity vs Reflectivity* implies that some individuals respond to new learning stimuli first and reflect later, while other individuals reflect first and respond afterwards. Although the latter might be intellectually sounder, the former has its uses in certain situations, and by those who are in a position to use intuitive knowledge.

To enable utilisation of styles of learning, Honey and Mumford (2000) designed a Learning Style Questionnaire (LSQ) which is widely used. The LSQ constitutes a self-assessment tool that indicates which style is generally utilised by the individual completing it. Four main uses of knowledge derived from the LSQ are:

- Increased awareness of learning activities that are congruent with the individual's learning style.
- A better choice of activities leading to more effective and economical learning.
- identification of areas in which an individual's less effective learning processes can be improved.
- Development of ways in which specific learning skills can be improved, for example reflective learning.

### Adapting to students' styles of learning

It is arguable that, where feasible, the mentor should endeavour to develop awareness of their mentee's learning style and approach to see if they can adapt to them to make their teaching more effective. This could make the achievement of practice objectives easier and more efficient.

An example of the adaptation of the *Theorists vs Pragmatists* style of learning is as follows. For instance, if the mentor finds that a particular student has leanings towards the pragmatist style, for any particular component of learning, that is, they immediately want to know how the learning applies to actual patient care situations, then the mentor can focus on the practical application of the learning first, moving on to related theories afterwards. The practical knowledge can follow immediately afterwards, and the theoretical knowledge later. Another student may wish to acquire all necessary theoretical knowledge before engaging in its practical application.

However, individual learning styles are not fixed, as the individual may consciously change their learning style according to the situation. Learners could in fact develop their ability in all styles of learning, and change or adapt them as new knowledge and skills are encountered. Style may also change through new experiences and at different stages of maturation.

## Approaches to learning

Evolving from different theories and styles, research has also identified different approaches to learning. Marton et al.'s (1997) research on approaches to learning identified individuals who take a deep approach to learning, those who take a surface approach and those who take the strategic approach. Students tend to use one of these three approaches. The defining features of each approach are presented in Box 2.4.

---

### Box 2.4    Deep, surface and strategic approaches to learning

| | |
|---|---|
| *Deep approach* | • Relates ideas to previous knowledge and experience<br>• Looks for patterns and underlying principles<br>• Checks evidence and relates it to conclusions<br>• Examines logic and argument cautiously and critically<br>• Engages with full interest with the course content |
| *Surface approach* | • Studies without reflecting on purpose and strategy<br>• Treats the course as unrelated bits of knowledge (discrete elements)<br>• Memorises facts and procedures in relation to assessments<br>• Finds difficulty in making sense of new ideas presented<br>• Feels undue pressure and worries about coursework |
| *Strategic approach* | • Puts consistent effort into studying<br>• Ensures conditions and materials for studying are appropriate<br>• Manages or organises time and effort to greatest effect<br>• Is alert to assessment requirements and criteria, and pays attention to cues about marking schemes<br>• Gears work to the perceived preferences of lecturers |

---

Whether a student takes the deep or surface approach to learning (Marton et al., 1997) might also depend on the stage of development of the subject area. Social sciences and arts may warrant a deep approach, while parts of science subjects such as biology and law might only require surface approaches, at least at earlier stages because they often constitute factual, single-answer knowledge. Newer and less factual subjects might also warrant a deep approach.

Approaches to learning also relate to the quality of the learning undertaken. Ramsden reports that if someone treated learning as an external imposition and concentrated on memorising facts, then that person was taking a surface approach to learning, and this would result in poor knowledge and understanding of the subject. Alternatively, 'if they intended to understand and interacted vigorously with the content of the text (a deep approach), they stood a better chance of getting the author's message and being able to remember the supporting facts' (1988: 19). As for adapting to the student's approach to learning, the mentor would prefer the student to take a deep approach but, during very busy times, strategic and surface approaches might temporarily be relevant.

## Principles of learning

Based on the views, theories, styles and approaches to learning discussed in this chapter, there are certain generally agreed principles of learning that can be deduced from them, which can make learning more effective, from both facilitators' and learners' standpoints. Mostly adapted from Davies (1982) and Knowles et al. (1998), these are:

- Whatever a student learns, they must actively learn for themselves – no one can learn it for them.
- Each student learns at their own chosen pace, as this varies depending on their particular circumstances, mental abilities and various other factors.
- A student learns more when each step is immediately reinforced or corrected.
- Full, rather than partial, mastery of each step makes the total more meaningful.
- When given responsibility for their own learning, the student is more highly motivated and likely to learn and retain more.
- The teacher as manager of learning should assume that McGregor's (1987) theory Y prevails, that is, learners are motivated to learn and seek out learning that is consistent with their practice objectives without being directed or coerced to do so.
- Students who come to education expecting to be passively fed information and knowledge should be eased into andragogical principles of learning and teaching soon after.

## Chapter Summary

This chapter has focused predominantly on the what and how of learning professional knowledge and competence. Having completed this chapter you will have learned about:

- What healthcare learners learn, and why, in the context of the student's learning needs in relation to knowledge and competence, and the different types of knowledge associated with professional skills.

- The definitions of competence and healthcare competencies, and issues related to them.
- Major views and perspectives on learning, teaching and education, which include what learning is, different perspectives on learning and where healthcare learners learn.
- Theories underpinning learning, in particular behaviourist learning theories (including Bandura's social learning theory), cognitive learning theories and humanistic learning theories such as andragogy and self-directed learning, the student-centred approach to learning and learning as self-actualisation.
- How learners learn healthcare skills. This included an examination of major styles of learning, and approaches to learning such as deep, surface and strategic learning. How the mentor could adapt their mentoring activities to students' styles and approaches to learning, and a brief on principles of learning.

# THREE

# Facilitating Learning

## Introduction

Having explored what mentoring, preceptoring and similar roles are, the reasons for these roles, and how they can be performed effectively, in Chapter 1, and then the different perspectives on learning, along with related theories and styles in Chapter 2, this chapter focuses on the teaching and learning facilitation role of the mentor. This chapter therefore covers:

- Whose learning healthcare practitioners facilitate, and what the reasons are for having to be able to do so.
- Whether we should teach or facilitate learning, what the two terms mean, and different approaches to teaching and learning.
- Different ways of facilitating learners' clinical skills acquisition.
- How to facilitate knowledge acquisition and how to plan a structured teaching session.
- The use of different teaching methods and teaching aids, and the advantages and disadvantages of each of them.
- Some of the issues related to facilitation of learning in clinical settings.

Over the years, both the UKCC and the NMC have identified the mentor as a 'teacher' in the clinical setting. The mentor's competence under the 'facilitation of learning' domain and the related outcomes identified by the NMC (2006a) were noted in Chapter 2 (Box 2.1).

## Chapter outcomes

On completion of this chapter, you should be able to:

1. Ascertain the full range of people whom healthcare practitioners teach.
2. Identify the reasons for teaching and facilitating learning, and the definitions and different perceptions of teaching.
3. Identify and explore the application of learning theories and styles.
4. Identify and apply the steps involved in effective planning for skills teaching and teaching knowledge base.
5. Explore different methods of teaching and presentation, and the use of different teaching aids.
6. Analyse some of the problems that might be encountered during the facilitation of learning.

## Whose Learning do Healthcare Practitioners Facilitate, and Why?

### Activity 3.1 – Who do healthcare professionals teach?

To start exploring facilitation of learning, first make a list of all groups of people who nurses and other healthcare professionals teach. Having done this, add the specific healthcare topics that they are likely to teach to the different groups of individuals.

The healthcare professional's role includes a substantial teaching component, and therefore you might have felt that Activity 3.1 was rather simplistic. It does however reflect the reality and, in response to the activity, you might have mentioned:

- Nurses teaching student nurses (first, second and third year), healthcare assistants on national vocational qualifications courses, patients/service users, patient's relatives, and junior doctors.
- Midwives teach women/service users, for example new mothers and fathers, how to look after a new baby.
- The practice nurse teaches primary (and secondary) level ill-health prevention, for example how to quit smoking, lose weight, expectant mothers regarding their diet, and relaxation for those with high blood pressure.
- SCPHNs teach mothers with different needs, such as single teenage mothers or those in different age groups.

### Why do healthcare professionals need to know how to facilitate learning?

On a day-to-day basis, the healthcare professional's role focuses largely on attending to patients' and service users' health problems. Teaching activities generally tend to be relegated to a more transient activity to be engaged in at opportune moments. Nevertheless, there are several reasons why healthcare professionals teach and facilitate learning. First, in addition to teaching colleagues and juniors being a job requirement for most healthcare professionals by virtue of their contract of employment, it also constitutes one of the four essential components of nursing and midwifery (Wright, 1990), the other components being clinical practice, care organisation and involvement in research. Correspondingly, the *NHS KSF* (DoH, 2004a: 57) notes under 'personal and people development' that healthcare professionals have to contribute to 'the development of others during ongoing work activities [by] structured approaches ... informal and ad hoc methods ...', and demonstrate and share skills and knowledge.

Similarly, teaching usually forms part of healthcare professionals' codes of practice, which stipulate that they must be willing to share skills and experience (NMC, 2007).

The previous NMC (2004a) *COPC* actually specified that the RN 'must … share [your] knowledge, skill and expertise with other members of the team as required for the benefit of patients and service users' (clause 4.3); and has 'a duty to facilitate students of nursing, midwifery and specialist community public health nursing and others to develop their competence' (clause 6.4). This form of teaching includes teaching new skills to colleagues (RNs/RMs), for example the use of new medical devices such as a new glucometer, how to conduct a patient assessment, the Doppler technique, and teaching learners.

Teaching is also an integral component of healthcare professionals' pre-registration programmes, as identified by the NMC's (2004b) standards of proficiency, for instance, and which therefore implies that the nurse will have acquired some teaching skills during their pre-registration programme. The outcomes related to 'teaching', stated under the domain personal and professional development for entry to the register, are: 'Enhance the professional development and safe practice of others through peer support, leadership, supervision and teaching', and

- Contribute to creating a climate conducive to learning.
- Contribute to the learning experiences and development of others by facilitating the mutual sharing of knowledge and experience.
- Demonstrate effective leadership in the establishment and maintenance of safe nursing practice.

Furthermore, specialist RNs and other healthcare professionals are at times required or invited to do small-group teaching on specific aspects of their specialist areas, within the healthcare trust, or classroom teaching on specialist university-based courses.

Additionally, healthcare professionals might also engage in teaching merely to advance the teaching or presentation skills that they have previously acquired to varying degrees. They can thereby also start to develop public-speaking skills. For more experienced mentors, teaching provides them with an opportunity to apply the principles of teaching and learning, and experiment with new teaching techniques. Furthermore, mentors have to teach because of variable levels of success in joint education-trust roles such as lecturer-practitioners, and the clinical teaching role of nurse lecturers.

## Facilitating Learning or Teaching?

At times we hear the statement, 'John (or Jane) is an excellent (or a born) teacher', but, as with most skills, teaching can be regarded as an 'art' and a 'science'. This means that although someone may appear to have a natural knack for teaching, it is also a skill that can be learned, using scientifically deduced theories. Short or long teaching courses such as the City and Guilds 7307 *Certificate in Teaching Adult Learners* course, or the *Post-graduate Certificate in Education*, are designed specifically for this purpose. After several years of teaching experience, eventually the skill becomes so well developed and refined that it appears akin to an artistic talent. However, thinking about some of the concepts discussed in Chapter 2, such as self-directed learning and reflective learning, consider the question 'Should mentors teach mentees and juniors, or facilitate their learning?' Both concepts are suggested for contemporary mentoring activities.

## Approaches to teaching and learning

Dictionaries tend to define teaching as 'to tell or show, to give instruction or lessons in' or 'to enable (a person) to do something by instruction and training'. Such definitions tend to signify teaching as one-way traffic, that is, the teacher controls the content, direction and flow of the session's content. It also reflects one of the earlier approaches to teaching, while Joyce et al. (2002) indicate that there are more than 22 models of teaching. Alternatively, Morton-Cooper and Wilkes (1993) state that there are three main approaches. These are:

1. Teaching can be seen as imparting knowledge and skills by the teacher who is the expert in the subject area, and the teacher selects and imparts pre-determined knowledge and skills to students, who in turn are passive recipients of the instruction. The approach may result in students acquiring knowledge but feeling inhibited from exploring alternatives.
2. Teaching as enabling active learning, in which the teacher structures learning activities for students so that they actively engage with the subject matter and explore specific topic areas in the curriculum or syllabus. Thus the teacher leads a student to conclusions by enquiry and questioning.
3. Teaching as facilitating learning, whereby teachers work in partnership with students and jointly determine their learning needs in the overall context of the curriculum, and the means by which those learning needs will be met. The teacher creates the conditions for learning and does not control all learning outcomes, thus allowing the student a substantial degree of choice in what to learn.

These three approaches identified by Morton-Cooper and Wilkes tend to reflect an evolving trend from the earlier (1) implying a teacher-centred approach, to (2) and (3) being much more learner centred, and therefore progressing from teaching to facilitation of learning. The approach chosen of course depends on several factors such as particular student groups, the teacher's own beliefs about teaching and learning, or a deliberate combination of these as the teacher feels appropriate.

The three teaching approaches can also be categorised as didactic, Socratic or facilitative respectively. In education generally, the trend has been very much to move away from teacher-centred approaches to student-centred ones. This was also advocated by Bruner (1960) whose 'discovery learning' theory suggests that learning is more effective when it is an active process stimulated through student curiosity. The teacher therefore devises situations, poses problems or questions, and creates the medium for the student to discover structures and principles underlying the situation or topic area. This approach feeds into problem-based learning, which entails an instructional method in which students work in small groups or individually to gain knowledge from simulated problem situations and acquire problem-solving skills at the same time.

Mentors can use these approaches in their learning facilitation roles. Problem-based learning can be implemented in the form of self-directed learning in clinical practice, in, for example, management of a staff conflict situation, management of a new illness or syndrome, the use of limited learning resources. The teacher must however ensure that the learning is directly linked to achieving learning objectives or competencies of the module or the course.

Current definitions of teaching take these evolving learning philosophies into account. For example, according to Curzon (2001: 21), 'Teaching is a system of activities intended to induce learning, comprising the deliberate and methodical creation and control of those conditions in which learning does occur.' The definition does not reflect teacher-centred one-way information giving.

*Teacher-centred or learner-centred approaches*
Teacher-centred teaching approaches clearly imply that the teacher directs the content of the teaching session. This may have advantages in being economical, in that with their deep knowledge of the subject the teacher can maximise the allocated time by selecting and focusing on the most significant areas of the topic.

Drawing on the theories underlying patient or service user-centred therapy for people with psychological problems, Rogers (1983) formulated the student-centred approach to learning, which formed a major landmark in approaches to teaching and learning. Rogers suggested that:

- Human beings have a natural potentiality for learning.
- Much significant learning is acquired through doing.
- Learning is facilitated when the student participates responsibly in the learning process.
- The most socially useful learning in the modern world is the learning of the process of learning, a continuing openness to experience and incorporation into oneself of the process of change.

## Activity 3.2 – Teacher-centred or student-centred teaching

To follow up the aforementioned approaches to teaching, identify a number of factors that you consider to be the strengths and weaknesses of teacher-centred and student-centred teaching methods, in healthcare professional education programmes.

Jarvis (1995) notes that using teacher-centred methods of teaching reinforces hierarchical social relationships between teachers and learners (or mentor and student), and thereby replicates models of authority in which the teacher might be seeking to control and mould individuals to fit into social systems. Rogers (1983) suggested earlier that such approaches cause learners to become dependent on teachers and thereby obstruct growth and development.

The possible weaknesses of teacher-centred methods or strategies include the following:

- They assume that students usually lack discipline and are irresponsible.
- They disregard experience as a resource for learning.
- The orientation to learning is subject-centred rather than building on individual students' existing knowledge.
- The motivation to learn is external, for example by passing courseworks.
- They can suppress the individual's creative powers.
- Students' opinions and questions tend to be largely overlooked.

Rogers sees the teacher as a facilitator of learning, a provider of resources for learning, and someone who shares feelings as well as knowledge with learners. Furthermore, he indicates that crucial to effective facilitation of learning is the relationship between individual learners and the facilitator. The prerequisites for being an effective facilitator of learning are awareness of self and being oneself in the teaching situation, that is, genuineness, trust and acceptance of students, and empathic understanding (as mentioned in Chapter 2):

- *Genuineness* – The facilitator portrays full honesty and willingness to declare their strengths and the areas in which they are lacking, where appropriate. They remain a real person and are not sucked into the image of a distant and authority-vested teacher.
- *Trust and acceptance* – The facilitator must be able to gain and retain the student's trust, and vice versa, and overtly accept any limitations students might have.
- *Empathic understanding* – The facilitator consistently endeavours to see situations from the learner's viewpoint.

Rogers contrasts the kind of learning that is concerned solely with cognitive functioning, for example acquiring knowledge, with that involving the whole person. The learning naturally needs to be guided by the approved curriculum of the course the student is on to be able to obtain the relevant award (i.e. qualification). Rogers suggests that it is possible for the teacher to build into a programme this freedom to learn. This can be done by using students' own experiences and problems so that relevance is obvious, and by identifying relevant resources for the students, both material and human. The goal of education is therefore to enable the student to become a fully functioning person (Rogers and Freiberg, 1994).

In healthcare learning, the student-centred approach is reflected in andragogy, but the latter needs to be tailored to individual students' responses to it. Facilitation of learning is also consistent with the andragogical approach to teaching and learning, as advocated by Knowles et al. (1998) (and discussed in Chapter 2) and with 'learning by insight', 'an unforeseen re-organisation by the learner of his field of experience' (Curzon, 2001: 88). A concept analysis of facilitation of learning by Cross (1996) revealed that the

- prerequisites of being a facilitator are the facilitator's qualities of realness, that is, caring and empathy, access to learning situations and the motivation of students and social influences;
- defining attributes of facilitation are a process of enabling change, a climate of learning which includes mutual trust, acceptance and respect, and the nature of interaction being student centred, negotiated and collaborative;
- consequences of facilitation are reciprocal change and feedback, and increased independence.

## Activity 3.3 – Mentoring Jane

Consider the following case study. Jane is a 34-year-old ex-schoolteacher who is now a first-year midwifery student. Jane is a graduate, who, after initial teacher training, soon found the job easy but had no wish to take on management responsibilities. The job was soon becoming too routine when she realised that in fact she had always wanted to be a midwife instead. Jane is also raising her own family and has remained an active member of the Parents and Teachers Association.

Consider the ways in which Jane's mentor, Julie, can take a learner-centred approach to learning facilitation during the practice placement. Make some notes taking into account Jane's previous vocation.

Mentors can consider ascertaining and adapting their facilitation of learning role to mentees' previous knowledge of health, their preferred styles and approaches to learning, as noted in Chapter 2. Jane's age, responsibility and discipline as a qualified teacher and a mother can be taken into account when taking a learner-centred approach to placement learning. A self-directed approach to learning in consultation with Julie can be warranted.

Despite these benefits of the student-centred approach to teaching, there could also be drawbacks, some of which are identified in Box 3.1.

---

**Box 3.1   Arguments for and criticisms of the learner-centred or person-centred approach to teaching**

*Arguments for:*

- Motivates, as aims and objectives are clear and relevant
- Learning is meaningful
- Encourages divergent and critical thinking through dialogue
- Allows autonomy and creativity

*Criticisms:*

- Can be time consuming if emphasis is on how much ground is covered, rather than the nature of learning that occurs (Rogers, 1983, was aware of this and suggested that there should be freedom within a system of constraints)
- Structure and guidelines may suffer
- Timetables and deadlines might not get adhered to
- Assumption that everyone engages in self-directed learning

---

Despite likely weaknesses, the student-centred approach to facilitation of learning is preferred as it entails more active involvement in learning. This is also consistent with old sayings such as, 'what we do we understand, what we see we remember, what we hear we forget' (Neary, 2000a: 93) and in relation to the senses and remembering, that we remember 90 per cent of all we do, 50 per cent of all we see, but only 10 per cent of all we hear.

In experiential learning, as a way of adapting learning theories to methods of teaching, students need to be given opportunities for 'doing', that is, applying or using the knowledge or skill. For example, most healthcare courses include the topic 'moving and handling patients'. This is an apt example that lends itself to experiential learning, in that having been exposed to the knowledge base (e.g. principles of moving and handling), students can then learn by doing. This can occur in university skills laboratories under close supervision of the facilitator. Students can be given problem situations to solve, which could enable them to make the topic their own and internalise it.

A concluding suggestion on facilitation of learning is that, in the context of the current-day vehement push towards efficiency, mentors and mentees need to seize learning opportunities as they arise, which is referred to as opportunistic learning or teachable moments.

## Facilitating Learners to Acquire Clinical Skills

Healthcare professions are skill-based vocations, which means that learning leads to becoming competent (or 'proficient' according to 'standards of proficiency' documents) at performing specific clinical interventions to improve patients' or service users' health. Competence was defined and discussed in Chapter 2. According to Curzon (2001), a skill signifies having expertise in an activity which has been developed as the result of training and/or experience, enabling the individual to perform the particular task with effectiveness and flexibility. It requires effective mind and muscle co-ordination, resulting in the production of appropriate, swift and meaningful patterns of movement. These are the distinguishing features of a 'skilled activity', which also include dexterity, the ability to respond quickly, spatial ability, and the capacity to share attention among a number of more or less simultaneous demands (Curzon, 2001). These definitions and features apply to healthcare clinical skills and competencies as well.

### Learning motor skills

Progression with learning and mastering clinical skills can be identified along a continuum that identifies early attempts at learning a skill to becoming proficient. A widely used framework for identifying levels of psychomotor skill development and testing in healthcare courses is that suggested by Steinaker and Bell (1979) in a taxonomy of experiential learning. The term *taxonomy* broadly refers here to levels of learning, that is, lower-level learning to higher levels. In Steinaker and Bell's model, skill development progresses from exposure, through participation, identification and internalisation to dissemination.

Experiential learning refers to learning that involves going through the experience of actually doing or engaging in the skill. Competency or skill development through the different levels occurs over the three-year course. The five levels and the likely interpretation (or criteria) related to a clinical skill are presented in Box 3.2.

---

### Box 3.2    Taxonomy levels and criteria

| Levels | Criteria |
|---|---|
| *Exposure* | • Have some knowledge of concepts, terms and methods used in clinical practice<br>• Show willingness to participate |
| *Participation* | • Interact well with patients/service users<br>• Carry out activities under supervision<br>• Explain activities when questioned |
| *Identification* | • Apply theory to practice<br>• Demonstrate awareness of situations<br>• Interpret information correctly<br>• Act on one's own without having to be prompted |
| *Internalisation* | • Consistently apply theory to practice in a range of settings<br>• Compare and contrast different approaches to practices<br>• Determine implications of practices<br>• Solve problems by analysis and evaluation<br>• Show willingness to share experiences |
| *Dissemination* | • Use opportunities to teach patients service users and families<br>• Share experiences with peers and others<br>• Accurately write and verbalise information about teaching and management issues |

---

Consider a mental health student who has to demonstrate a certain level of proficiency in helping or counselling skills by the end of their third year of professional education:

1. *Exposure* – refers to the student observing the mentor helping or counselling appropriate service users and becoming aware of the pre-conditions and specific helping skills being used by the mentor.
2. *Participation* – refers to when, under mentor supervision, the student attempts to use selected helping skills.
3. *Identification* – is when the student starts to feel competent at some of the helping skills, and this is acknowledged by their mentor.
4. *Internalisation* – can be difficult to achieve within the constraints of the pre-registration course, as this implies that the learner is so proficient at these skills that they see them as part of themselves as a person.
5. *Dissemination* – refers to being so knowledgeable and competent in a skill that the person can have specific and valid opinions about the skill, can explain them, and even teach them, which is difficult to achieve in a pre-registration course.

To teach competencies at the appropriate level entails careful planning that determines the teacher's approach, student behaviour and assessment techniques. Another well-established model of learning a clinical skill is Benner's (2001) stages of skill acquisition, which is based on a framework initially developed by Dreyfus and Dreyfus (1980). These stages are novice, advanced beginner, competent, proficient and expert, in this sequence, and they relate to longer-term activities on expertise development as they progress from initial cruder attempts to more refined performance with a substantial associated knowledge base.

Fitts and Posner (1973) earlier suggested that there are three phases of learning a skill: the cognitive phase, associative phase and autonomous phase:

1. *Cognitive phase* – concerned with the learning of the procedure, but the more complex the skill, the longer the learning will take.
2. *Associative phase* – engaging in skilled performance of part-skills or in whole practical skills, and interfering responses are eliminated.
3. *Autonomous phase* – the skill becomes automatic and can be performed without the student thinking much about it.

The three phases are not completely distinct; as they overlap, with one phase leading to the next.

## Teaching psychomotor skills

A major component of the mentor's role is to teach clinical skills. Various aspects need to be considered in relation to this.

### Activity 3.4 – Skill acquisition and maintenance

Think of, and list all factors that a teacher needs to consider, and all preparations that they need to make to teach a particular clinical skill. Then list all factors that might affect efficient acquisition of the psychomotor skill in the clinical area. Finally list all factors that might affect maintenance and performance of the clinical skill at the same or higher standard in the clinical area.

There are several factors that need to be considered when preparing to teach a clinical skill. Those required for teaching blood glucose monitoring, for instance, include:

- which patient?
- condition requiring it; area/patient;
- equipment needed;
- procedure for taking a blood sample;
- gain patient's consent;
- factors affecting reading of results;
- ensure there's enough blood on the test strip;
- safety aspects;
- own knowledge;
- the student's knowledge base – practical and theoretical;

- result – up/down/normal;
- opportunities to practise;
- frequency of measurement;
- testing the equipment and cleaning it after use;
- evaluate, observe, supervise;
- what if !!
- time allocated;
- how to record competence.

A list of factors that need to be considered for a particular clinical activity like the one above is rarely fully prescriptive as there are other variables that need to be taken into account in relation to the individual patient's health problems or needs, and the equipment and other resources that are available.

Teaching a clinical skill requires first of all a skills analysis. Generally, the trust's procedure for the skill constitutes a very good basis for structuring a lesson plan for the skill. The mentor can also consider how the task is performed or executed, step by step, by those who are recognised as consti at that skill. These are discussed shortly. Such a detailed analysis of the clinical skill constitutes its performance criteria, which is discussed in Chapter 6. Box 3.3 presents a set of principles of teaching a skill or competency that stands the test of time (extracted from Curzon, 2001). These are generally fully used when teaching a skill in the HEI's skills laboratory, but can be easily adapted by the mentor when teaching in the clinical setting.

---

**Box 3.3  Principles of teaching a skill or competency**

1. *Initially demonstrate the skill in its entirety as a fully integrated set and cycle of operations.* The demonstration needs to be accompanied by a clear step-by-step commentary, and it must be a demonstration of mastery of the skill. The correct movements that go to make up the skill must be in evidence from the outset.
2. *Break the skill down into its component and subordinate activities.* Each action must be demonstrated, explained, and analysed. The relation of separate activities to one another, and their integration into a hierarchy of sequences that make up the skill must be stressed.
3. *Skill acquisition lessons require supervised, reinforced, and carefully spaced practice by students.* It is only by experiencing and repeating the essential movements that the learner can discover the kinaesthetic cues of successful performance.
4. *Continuous, swift and accurate feedback must be provided for the learner.* Delayed feedback on performance makes the feedback less effective.
5. *Assess part-skills or the whole skill regularly and in realistic conditions.* Evidence should also be sought on the ability of the student to transfer the acquired skill to related situations.
6. *Achievement of competence at one level ought to be accepted as a necessary preparation for moving to higher level of skill.* The learner should be able to progress from competent performance to proficient, and so on.

*Source*: adapted from Curzon (2001).

---

The principles presented in Box 3.3 constitute a firm foundation for developing a skill-teaching session. Drawing on this, and on healthcare professionals' perceptions of factors that need to be considered when preparing to teach a psychomotor skill, the teacher should also consider taking the following actions before the actual skill-teaching session.

- Practise the skill yourself, using the relevant procedures and equipment.
- Ensure that, as teacher, you are up to date on grounds of evidence-based practice.
- Have all equipment and materials ready.
- Arrange for your learner(s) to hear and see.
- State the aim of the session.
- Show the finished product if possible.
- Ask the student/patient to verbalise the action.
- Let the student/patient practise the skill.

### Domains of learning and levels of skill acquisition

Exactly what do healthcare students learn on their pre-registration courses? They learn knowledge and competence related to healthcare interventions. Each intervention comprises three domains of activity: psychomotor, cognitive and affective (e.g. Bloom, 1956; Girot, 1993). The psychomotor domain refers to muscular and motor skills; the cognitive domain refers to the use of knowledge and information; and the affective domain refers to attitudes, emotions and values. The three domains broadly equate with skills, knowledge and attitudes, which largely further equate with doing, thinking and feeling respectively. The three domains are integrated essential components of each competency, and not necessarily distinct and separate activities. All healthcare interventions incorporate these three domains, and therefore learning the clinical skill must also incorporate all three components.

---

 **Think Point 3.1 – Psychomotor, cognitive and affective domains of competencies**

Consider any two clinical interventions (e.g. blood pressure taking, counselling or ward management) to ascertain whether each contains all three components: skill, knowledge and attitude.

---

The sequence of events that both teacher and learner should engage in during skill acquisition is summarised in Table 3.1. It captures the principles of teaching and facilitation of learning of a psychomotor skill or competency that incorporates the cognitive and affective domains. The five components of the affective domain to be achieved by the learner are *receiving, responding, valuing, organising* and *characterising* (Davies, 1982; Krathwold et al., 1964).

After practising the skill on several occasions, a summative assessment of competence will be performed by the mentor, and the learner is usually permitted to

**Table 3.1 Skills teaching sequence**

| Psychomotor domain | Cognitive domain | Affective domain |
|---|---|---|
| *Awareness* that learner lacks the skill or is deficient in it | Establish existing related knowledge base | *Receiving* – i.e. realising that it will be beneficial to learn the skill |
| Ensure the learner is *motivated* to learn the skill | Be active in seeking related knowledge | *Responding* – is willing, and takes action to learn the skill |
| *Analysis* of the step-by-step procedure/components of the skill | Having clear objectives in learning it, of possible sources of learning | Learner appreciates the step-by-step procedure, the materials required |
| *Prepare* equipment, etc., to teach it | Assemble appropriate equipment/devices and materials | |
| *Demonstrate* the skill at normal speed | Learner observes and concentrates on all details of the procedure | |
| *Discuss* each step just performed; *re-demonstrate* part-skills as required | State rationale for each action; emphasise important points; discuss safety points; encourage learner to ask questions | *Valuing* – the rationales for each step taken. Learner is willing to participate in performing the skill or part-skill. |
| Allow learner to *perform* whole skill/part-skills | Select components to work on, and actually 'doing' the skill, i.e. experiencing it | *Organising* – mental rehearsal of each skill component; asking questions |
| Allow to *perform* the skill under supervision | Observe in silence | |
| *Praise and review* | Give feedback on performance Reward progress Correct any mistakes | Reinforcement and sense of achievement, confidence |
| Allow to apply/repeat the skill under supervision | Using the learning in real situations. Assess progress and knowledge of rationales | *Characterising* – accepting the agreed protocol is the correct way of performing the skill |

practise without direct supervision. One of the key purposes of Table 3.1 is to highlight how the cognitive and affective domains of learning are integral components of learning any clinical intervention. It involves taking a holistic approach and being aware of how the patient feels at all times during the activity.

As a general guide, 25 per cent of the lesson time should be used to demonstrate the skill, 15 per cent in verbal explanation, and 60 per cent for guided practice. So, for effective acquisition of the skill or competency, it is important to consider the requirements for effective teaching. Other factors that affect effective and efficient acquisition of the skill include:

- the complexity of the skill;
- individual differences in speed of learning, or background;
- its transferability to real-life settings;
- teaching situation – environment, light, space, room temperature;
- the quality of instruction;
- knowledge of progress;
- availability of practice opportunities;
- availability of necessary equipment – checking them beforehand, describing them;
- getting feedback on skill performance;
- a positive approach;
- a running commentary if appropriate;
- a true-to-life setting;
- allowing time for discussion;
- time for practice – with positive reinforcement.

The types of knowledge associated with skills teaching is practical knowledge (i.e. 'knowing how') and theoretical knowledge (i.e. more in-depth 'knowing that'). Healthcare courses involve acquisition of both types of knowledge, and students are assessed on them at different academic levels, as detailed shortly in this chapter.

## Facilitating Knowledge Acquisition

Despite the current paradigm shift away from teaching to facilitation of learning, formal teaching also has its place in professional preparatory programmes. Many clinical skills and knowledge components are best imparted to learners through teaching. There will be times when the mentor will have to conduct short structured teaching sessions, probably in a room in the clinical setting that can be used for this purpose. These sessions could be quite short or last an hour or more, delivered to a small group of learners or colleagues. Therefore a good insight into how to structure and deliver a teaching session is a useful component of the mentor's armoury of capabilities.

Effective teaching requires careful and thorough planning. The lesson needs to be structured fully, with flexibility built in depending on whether it is being delivered to a large group, or to smaller group workshops.

### Planning a structured teaching session

Logical sequencing of a structured teaching session constitutes lesson planning, an example of which is presented in Box 3.4.

---

Box 3.4   Steps in lesson planning

1.  Identify the topic of the lesson
2.  Research the subject
3.  Consider the students in relation to their existing knowledge
4.  Write down the aims and objectives
5.  Jot down as many points as possible in keeping with the objectives, then select, prune, sequence and structure these points
6.  Select the appropriate teaching methods
7.  Screen the activities against the objectives
8.  Write the lesson (include teaching aids)
9.  Prepare aids, equipment and classroom
10. Give the lesson
11. Evaluate the lesson

---

Each step presented in Box 3.4 requires specific attention in its own right. For instance, the third step requires the teacher to consider the students in relation to the knowledge they already have, as well as any prior reading that was required or suggested before the teaching session. This accords with the use of appropriate learning theories such as Ausubel et al.'s (1978) assimilation theory (discussed in Chapter 2). It is also consistent with Bruner's (1960) notion of linking new learning to previous knowledge.

As to the sequencing of lesson content (step 5 in Box 3.4), the Herbartian rule (Quinn and Hughes, 2007: 20) of sequence (or 'sequence procedures') for lesson presentation has stood the test of time and is also referred to as traditional rule. It involves proceeding from:

1.  *The known to the unknown* – link new concepts to what is already known (e.g. water to blood, water pipes to blood vessels).
2.  *The simple to the complex* – simple explanations to more complex areas; increasing level of complexity (e.g. diffusion in a jar to movement of oxygen and Co2 between alveoli and alveolar capillaries; intra- and extra-cellular movement of potassium).
3.  *The concrete to the abstract* – demonstrable visible components to invisible concepts (e.g. aspirates or infusion to acidity vs alkalinity).
4.  *The particular to the general* – use specific examples to illustrate general theories (e.g. giving information reduces anxiety, people generally having a need to know what is happening).
5.  *Observation to reasoning* – from how things are done to why.
6.  *The whole view to the parts, then return to the whole view* – the subject matter as an entity, analysis of component parts, return to the overall view.

Step 6 in Box 3.4 suggests selecting the appropriate teaching methods. A range of teaching methods is available to the teacher (see Box 3.5). The teaching method(s) selected for the session must be based on principles of teaching and on learning theories. The appropriateness of the method depends on the teacher's level of knowledge of theories and principles and their values, research and verbal skills, facilitative skills, on the aims of the lesson, for instance.

---

### Box 3.5    Most frequently used teaching methods

- Lectures
- Buzz groups/work in sub-groups
- Seminars
- Skills demonstration
- Guided study and open learning
- Role plays
- Problem-solving games/exercises/ workshops
- Case study/patient-centred discussions

- Video recording a presentation
- Tutorial – individual/small group
- Ideas free-flow exercises (previously known as brainstorming)
- Questions and answers
- Formal lessons
- E-learning and distance learning
- Group discussion
- Team teaching

---

Each of these methods has its advantages and disadvantages which are examined later in this chapter. The eighth step in Box 3.4 is to 'write the lesson', and includes identifying the teaching aids to be used. An examples of a lesson plan is presented in Box 3.6.

---

### Box 3.6    Lesson or session plan

Date: ………..…..    Cohort: ………………    No of students:……………......…

Title of the course/module: …………………………..

Subject of lesson: …………………………………………

Duration of lesson: ………………………… (e.g. 1 hour)    Classroom: ………

Lesson/session aims:

Lesson/session learning outcomes:

Equipment/materials required:

| Time | Lesson content | Method | Teaching aids |
|------|----------------|--------|---------------|
| 5 mins | Testing previous lesson | Q & A | – |
| 2 mins | State and explain lesson objective | Verbal exposition | OPT |
| 15 mins | Concept I | Verbal exposition; Q & A | Whiteboard/flipchart |
| 15 mins | Concept II | Verbal exposition; discussion | Whiteboard/flipchart |
| 15 mins | Concept III | Verbal exposition; discussion | |
| 3 mins | Recapitulation | Verbal exposition | OPT |
| 4 mins | Test and evaluation | Q & A | OPT |
| 1 min | Announce title of next lesson | Verbal exposition | Whiteboard/flipchart |

Q & A = Questions and answers
OPT = Overhead projector and transparencies

---

In relation to steps 8 and 9, or the use of an appropriate range of teaching aids such as whiteboard/flipchart or OPTs, some of these will be explained briefly, and their advantages and disadvantages will also be explored later in this chapter.

In planning the lesson, the teacher needs to consider likely constraints such as class size (for instance is it 10 students or 200?), the number of pages of handouts if any given and availability of articles to be recommended. The teacher's aim in a lesson is to motivate, stimulate and communicate, to hold the class's attention and to achieve the defined objectives (Curzon, 2001), and therefore further essential considerations by the presenter are that:

1. The lesson must be pitched appropriately.
2. The teaching objectives must be realistic and clear.
3. Exposition must be ordered, simple and clear.
4. Development must be logical and consequential (flows coherently).
5. Presentation must be based on the essential 'social character' of the lesson (e.g. laboratory work or lecture).
6. Presentation must involve a variety of media.
7. Presentation must be related carefully to fluctuations in class attention.
8. Appropriate body language should be used.

Furthermore, a well-constituted presentation requires a clearly defined structure, the elements of which will normally include:

- An introduction, main part and conclusion.
- A logical sequence within each of the three parts.
- Regular sign-posting – this is where we have been, where we are now, and where we are about to go.
- Key learning points or main headings.
- Built-in monitoring and review – checking that the main learning points are being understood.

Appropriate communication and delivery skills are crucial. The presenter's role is also to engage with the audience, to challenge, to enthuse, to support, to motivate and to clarify. The next step is to give the lesson based on the lesson plan, and at the end of the lesson to evaluate it. The evaluation of the lesson can include use of an evaluation form, or to ask students to write three things, they liked or found most useful about the session, aspects that can be seen as weaknesses, and suggestions for improvement.

### Levels of theory acquisition

The objective of many a teaching session is to impart knowledge and understanding of the designated topic area and, depending on various factors, it can cover application, analysis and synthesis. These concepts are largely enshrined in the cognitive domain of Bloom's (1956) taxonomy of learning, which follows six hierarchical levels. The first or lower level of learning is the acquisition of knowledge, followed by the higher levels – comprehension, application, analysis, synthesis and evaluation, as illustrated here:

- *Knowledge* – refers to knowledge of topic area and content.
- *Comprehension* – refers to knowledge and comprehension.

- *Application* – refers to knowledge and comprehension, and application of concepts to general and specific settings.
- *Analysis* – refers to knowledge, comprehension, application and analysis of each concept.
- *Synthesis* – refers to knowledge, comprehension, application, analysis and synthesis.
- *Evaluation* – refers to knowledge, comprehension, application, analysis, synthesis and evaluation.

*Knowledge* is the most basic level of learning, in which the student shows recall of specific facts, classifications, categories, and sequences or methods in the topic area. It is a significant component of student assessment, as when the student has to demonstrate knowledge of human biology or of research methods. *Comprehension* refers to understanding and interpretation of the topic area, and can be shown by the student explaining theories and reasoning in their own words. It answers the question 'why' certain things happen or certain actions are taken, and the possible implications and consequences of these. *Application* occurs when the student applies knowledge and understanding to 'real-life' situations such as patient care. *Analysis* entails the ability to break down theories and concepts into their component parts, and explain the relationships between elements and the whole. It considers strengths and weaknesses, and separates the important aspects of information from the less important ones. *Synthesis* requires the individual to recombine various components of the topic area into a newly reconstructed whole. The student thereby utilises creativity in producing something unique, for example a plan, a design or a proposal. *Evaluation* implies the ability to make judgements regarding the value of material learned.

A simple and brief example of levels of learning related to 'the heart and blood pressure' is presented here to illustrate how cognitive levels of learning (Bloom, 1956) apply to learning in healthcare:

- *Knowledge* – knowing the anatomy and physiology of the heart and that pressure is exerted on the blood vessels each time the heart pumps a certain volume of blood through them.
- *Comprehension* – understanding that the reason for the heart beating rhythmically at approximately 60 beats every minute, generating a blood pressure (BP) of approximately 110/70 mm Hg is to ensure that essential ingredients such as glucose and oxygen are transferred to every tissue in the human body, and continuously.
- *Application* – awareness that the above BP reading can change for a variety of reasons, which might include diseased organs, and its significance for patient care.
- *Analysis* – when a person is seen to have high BP, the nurse needs to consider the whole range of reasons for this.
- *Synthesis* – designing, and advising the individual on, a set of actions to take to reduce their BP, and explaining the effects of unstable or high BP based on their unique aetiology and perceptions of high BP.
- *Evaluation* – ascertaining the value of the above set of actions, the skills and compliance of the patient in relation to them.

The analysis of the cognitive domain of learning is essential as it involves critical analysis, which as already noted above entails breaking down information, exploring relationships between elements, or organisation and structure of information. Critical analysis involves the use of critical thinking, whereby we:

- Examine all the component parts of a situation.
- Identify what existing knowledge or information we have, related to the situation.
- Distinguish relevant information from irrelevant.
- Challenge generalisations, assumptions and rituals.
- Imagine and explore alternatives and choose appropriate options.

Gopee (2002b) discusses an effective way in which students can demonstrate critical analysis in their written assignments. Furthermore, more recently, Krathwohl (2002) has suggested a refinement of Bloom's (1956) level of knowledge acquisition by suggesting that the sequence be represented as follows:

1 Remember → 2 Understand → 3 Apply → 4 Analyse → 5 Evaluate → 6 Create

The fifth and sixth levels are reversed, but, as with any new framework, it requires researching to ascertain its applicability.

## Teaching Methods and Teaching Aids

As discussed in the preceding section, skill demonstration is an effective way of teaching how to perform a professional skill. For structured lessons, effective teaching requires choosing and applying the appropriate teaching methods and aids, which are selected based on such factors as class size, aims of session, the students' existing knowledge levels, and so on. The most frequently used teaching methods were identified in Box 3.5.

### Teaching methods – their advantages and disadvantages

Lectures remain an efficient teaching method for imparting knowledge and comprehension of a selected section of a subject area. A lecture is economical in that the knowledge can be imparted to hundreds of students by one lecturer during a particular teaching session. In fact, the lecture can be televised live to other lecture theatres in the same or other universities, even in other countries.

However, only a limited level of application and analysis can be achieved, as it is difficult for each individual student to verbalise their views and other perspectives in very large groups. Moreover, it is easier for students oto let their minds wander off the subject, which they generally can't do in smaller groups. Discussions, workshops and groupwork to explore application, analysis and synthesis of components of the lecture should therefore always follow lectures. Similarly, the advantages and disadvantages of other teaching methods also need to be appreciated.

> ### Optional activity – Teaching methods: advantages and disadvantages
>
> Taking an analytical approach, the strengths and weaknesses of each of the examples of different teaching methods listed in Box 3.5 can be identified. Consider these different teaching methods, and feel free to add others of your own, and identify as many advantages and disadvantages as you can for each of these methods.

You should have been able to identify one or two advantages and disadvantages of each of the aforementioned teaching methods. With *skill demonstration,* for instance, the advantages include visual display of the skill being performed. It reinforces previously acquired knowledge of the skill, activates many senses, enables procedure-directed practice, correlates theory and practice and is economical on time. The disadvantages could be that the learner might be left/right-handed related to positioning of equipment, the skill might involve movements that are too complex, and too much information might be given. As learning and mastering a skill takes time, there is also a danger that the learner might be expected to perform the demonstrated skill at similar speed to the skilled demonstrator too soon.

The advantages of using *case studies* or *patient-centred discussions* as a teaching method are that there is active participation by students, that they are useful in the application of theory to practice, and that they present an opportunity for structured problem solving. This increases understanding of the situation, diagnosing the problem, creating alternative solutions and predicting outcomes or implications. The disadvantages could include insufficient patient data.

## Presentation and teaching aids

There are several types of presentation aids that the teacher can utilise to vary the session, and thereby to retain the audience's attention or to add emphasis to aspects of the session. These aids include:

- overhead projector and transparencies;
- flipchart and pens;
- whiteboard;
- Powerpoint presentations;
- showing video-cassette or DVD recordings;
- slides;
- models/objects;
- gapped handouts;
- simulated materials or liquids.

The purpose of teaching aids is therefore to introduce variety into the teaching process, to extend sensory perception, to extend visual perception, to give meaning to abstractions, and to assist in conceptualisation of complicated issues. The choice of visual aids involves consideration of appropriateness to the context or message, its cost effectiveness, its availability, and its suitability for your style of presentation. Each teaching aid requires a good understanding of how it works.

## Activity 3.5 – Strengths and weaknesses of different teaching aids

Consider the strengths and weaknesses of the different teaching aids listed earlier, add other ones that you know of, and discuss with someone who has had some experience of classroom teaching what might be the strengths and weaknesses of each of these aids.

The *Powerpoint presentation* is a highly favoured method of presenting the knowledge base of a topic area to small or large audiences. The advantage is that it is prepared in advance and can be made very lively and colourful with pictures, cartoons, and short films for more impact. The likely disadvantage might be that too many words are inserted in each slide, or if the slides are presented at a high speed this may not allow time for the audience to take the content in properly, or the equipment may fail (computers are known to explode).

## Issues with Facilitation of Learning in the Clinical Setting

The mentor's role includes teaching mentees on a one-to-one basis, and at times in small groups in the clinical setting. In both situations the mentor needs to have a clear view of various components of the session, for example the content and sequence of the presentation, to ensure the learner gains an orderly, systematic understanding of the topic or clinical skill. However, the problematic situations that might arise when facilitating student learning may present as challenges to the mentor.

For instance, there can be confusion in the interpretation of students' 'supernumerary status' during placements, in that the student may claim that they are there only to observe clinical activity, while the mentor believes they should observe and participate. Supernumerary status can be manipulated by some students to the extent that they take excessive time off clinical settings as study time, to the detriment of learning hands-on care and clinical skills, as many mentors claim that healthcare delivery is learned by doing, not by merely knowing about it. Perceptions of how to record reflective write-ups may vary.

Differences of views or interpretation of rules need to be resolved by discussion and consulting appropriate educational or trust personnel for further guidance.

In facilitation of learning there can be differences in perception of what a reflective write-up is, how many words it should contain, and whether to support arguments with references. In opportunistic learning, negotiating access to opportunities is a skill in its own right.

## Chapter Summary

This chapter has focused on the mentor's role in facilitation of learning, both formal and informal. Having completed this chapter you will have learned about:

- Whose learning healthcare practitioners facilitate, and why, and the various reasons for teaching, the definitions and different perceptions of teaching, along with why healthcare practitioners need to know how to facilitate learning.
- General perspectives on learning, indicating a move away from teaching to the notion of facilitating learning. Approaches to teaching and learning including teacher-centred methods, their uses and likely weaknesses, and the student-centred approach, which includes teaching styles and applying learning theories and styles. The movement comprises shifting away from formal teaching to much more learner-centred facilitation of learning.
- Facilitating learners to acquire clinical skills, teaching a psychomotor skill, the domains of learning, levels of psychomotor skills, and stages of skill acquisition.
- Facilitating knowledge acquisition, including undertaking planned and structured short teaching sessions, either at one-to-one level, or in small groups of learners.
- The types of knowledge associated with skills, such as practical knowledge and theoretical knowledge, along with levels of theory acquisition and levels and stages of skill acquisition (taxonomy levels).
- Step-by-step planning of teaching sessions, including utilisation of different methods of teaching, and teaching aids, and an analysis of how they can be used effectively.
- Some of the issues that might surface in facilitation of learning in the clinical setting.

# FOUR

# The Clinical Setting as an Effective Learning Environment

## Introduction

Having explored the concept of mentorship in Chapter 1, perspectives, theories and styles of learning in Chapter 2, and facilitation of learning in Chapter 3, this chapter focuses on the factors that make clinical settings effective learning environments. This chapter therefore covers:

- The reasons for requiring practice placements for students on healthcare professional education programmes, and then students' own perspectives, hopes and expectations before the start of placements.
- What a learning environment is, how to create and maintain a functional learning ethos in the clinical setting, and educational audit of practice placement settings.
- Utilisation of learning pathways, and guidelines, policies and standards for learning environments.
- Work-based learning, identifying and analysing what it is.
- What makes a clinical setting a learning organisation.
- Issues related to practice placements, and how they can be resolved.

Ensuring that the clinical setting is a learning environment is a key role of the mentor, according to research (e.g. Darling, 1984; Phillips et al., 2000). Under the domain 'creating an environment for learning' the NMC (2006a: 53) indicates that the mentor should be competent in creating 'an environment for learning, where practice is valued and developed, that provides appropriate professional and inter-professional learning opportunities and support for learning to maximise achievement for individuals'. Similar standards and guidelines were previously developed by the ENB (1997) under 'practice experience'.

Other aspects related to learning environments are identified under the domain 'context of practice', and include educational policies and managing change.

## Chapter outcomes

On completion of this chapter you should be able to:

1. Clearly identify students' perspectives and expectations of practice placements, and the clinical experiences that meet their learning needs.
2. Identify how a learning ethos can be created and maintained in the clinical setting, including research findings, inter-professional learning, and annual education audits as components.
3. Identify the benefits of work-based learning as a concept and activity in its own right, and the associated issues.
4. Identify how clinical settings can become learning organisations.
5. Recognise the likely problematic aspects related to practice placements, such as with integration of theory and practice and supernumerary status, and possible solutions to them.

## Learners on Practice Placements

This section of the chapter explores why practice placements are required, and students' perspectives, hopes and expectations in relation to practice objectives and clinical experiences during placements.

### The requirement for practice placements

The key reasons for clinical settings having to be learning environments for student practice placements are as follows. First, healthcare professions comprise skill or competency-based activities, and these skills are acquired predominantly in clinical settings. Several hundred student nurses, numerous AHP and medical students start their pre-registration or pre-service courses each year, and each student requires practice placements in clinical settings to learn patient care skills directly, or to consolidate and extend their learning from university skills laboratories. Most suitable clinical settings in the local trusts and the independent sector are used for placements, and the placement of all these students is arranged by the education institution's placement department. Each clinical setting is advised in advance of which students are starting on placement with them, and when. Students arrive on placement with a set of practice competencies to be achieved during the placement, which need to be planned in accordance with the specialist clinical skills and knowledge the particular setting offers.

Furthermore, the NMC's (2006a) competence for mentors under 'creating an environment for learning' comprises the following outcomes:

- Support students to identify both learning needs and experiences that are appropriate to their level of learning.
- Use a range of learning experiences, involving patients, clients, carers and the professional team, to meet defined learning needs.
- Identify aspects of the learning environment which could be enhanced, negotiating with others to make appropriate changes.
- Act as a resource to facilitate personal and professional development of others.

Another reason for clinical settings needing to be learning environments is the increasingly popular concept of work-based learning (discussed later in this chapter), which clearly recognises the wide occurrence and value of learning in clinical settings. However, various research studies have in the past revealed weaknesses of clinical settings as learning environments. Consequently, for learning to occur, the clinical setting must embody an ethos that nurtures and supports learning, but not deters.

## Students' perspectives, hopes and expectations

A number of clinical settings have an established welcome and orientation programmes for students starting practice placement with them, and an induction pack with specific clinical objectives for qualified new healthcare professionals. A named mentor is allocated to each student prior to the start of the placement, along with associate mentors. Both the mentor and the mentee have certain hopes and expectations of each other. So what does the student anticipate encountering at the start of the placement?

### Activity 4.1 – Student expectations from the placement

Your work base clearly has a wide range of specific knowledge and competence to offer learners during practice placements. From your experience of having students on placement, make some notes on what you feel are the expectations that students might have on starting placement in your clinical setting.

In addition to students' expectations, the staff in the clinical setting naturally also have certain expectations of students. They hope the student will be punctual, make every effort to integrate with the team, and be open-minded about the way care is delivered in the particular clinical setting. The mentor might expect the student to seek out learning experiences and opportunities, and ask questions about aspects that they do not understand. Box 4.1 lists some of the characteristics of 'good' learners.

---

**Box 4.1   Significant characteristics of learners for effective learning**

- Keen, enthusiastic and motivated to learn
- Open-minded
- Identifies own learning needs
- Open to feedback and constructive criticism
- Punctual
- Reflects on experiences

- Knows own limitations
- Able to adapt to different clinical settings
- Does not have negative thoughts prior to start of placement
- Utilises learning opportunities
- Communicates effectively
- Wants to self-improve
- Reads round the subject area

---

*Advanced preparation of learners*
Students find it useful if, prior to the practice placement, the clinical setting sends out a welcome letter, and even asks the student to come for an informal pre-placement

visit. It is useful if the student can also be advised of any recommended preparatory reading related to the clinical specialism. This action is in line with Ausubel et al.'s (1978) concept of 'advanced organiser', which signifies that learning is likely to occur more effectively if new experiences are linked to prior knowledge.

The value of communication prior to the beginning of the placement is that the student begins to become familiar with the clinical setting, gets to know more about the clinical specialism, meets the mentor, and staff get to know the student as well. The aim of this would be to ensure that the clinical experiences the student will encounter meet their learning needs and enable the achievement of their practice objectives.

## Creating and Maintaining a Learning Ethos in the Clinical Setting

Healthcare students acquire knowledge and competence in universities which are seen as well-established learning environments. The value of work-based learning (WBL) in enabling healthcare practitioners to achieve fitness to practise was referred to briefly in Chapter 1. However, to what extent are clinical settings learning environments?

### Activity 4.2 – A learning ethos in the clinical area

Using your current and past experience of factors that are significant in creating an effective learning experience for students during practice placements, make notes on the following. Who are the key people who are role models for learners (pre- and post-registration, others) in clinical settings? What are the factors that are important for the creation of a positive learning environment (including research-based factors) for everyone within any particular clinical setting?

To be a role model for anyone can be a sobering prospect for most people. In response to who the role models in clinical settings are, you would have identified a range of qualified healthcare professionals and probably even some unqualified staff involved in practice-based learning, including:

- everyone acting as a mentor;
- ward sisters/charge nurses;
- team leaders;
- specialist nurses (e.g. pain specialists);
- practice educators;
- other RNs on paybands 5 to 8;
- other healthcare professionals (e.g. physiotherapists, occupational therapists);
- tutors;
- other students;

- senior doctors, mainly consultants;
- outreach workers;
- clinical managers;
- healthcare assistants for specific skills;
- everyone who works in the clinical area.

The concept of role models was examined in Chapter 1.

## Clinical settings as learning environments

In response to Activity 4.2, that is, identifying the factors that are important for the creation of a positive learning environment, you might have noted friendly staff, positive attitude and allocated time for teaching. Good communication is of course essential, as is the learner feeling that they are part of the team. Team members with up-to-date knowledge of the latest research in their specialism generally make a positive impression. The availability and accessibility of research literature in the working environment, stocked in a learning resources section or in a resource room, also creates a positive image.

Furthermore, you might have noted that staff showing some awareness of students' likely learning needs and their stage of knowledge and competence development also create positive impressions. The enthusiasm of team members with responsibility for teaching in clinical settings, and practice educators' input, generate impetus for learning. Constructive comments on skill performance in an appropriate environment is usually appreciated by learners. A culture in which clinical staff are open to new ideas and share new learning from courses also presents healthy perspectives, as does good staff morale.

In an early study of clinical learning environments, Fretwell (1980) aimed to find out:

- Whether students felt they needed teaching in the ward environment.
- The attitudes of trained staff and learners as to the amount of teaching that might be needed.
- Who should teach.

In conclusion, Fretwell identified the key components of the 'ideal learning environment' as anti-hierarchy, teamwork, negotiation, communication and availability of trained nurses for responding to students' questions.

The first aim of the study was to explore whether student nurses felt they needed teaching in the ward environment – because in the 1980s nursing students were rostered and salaried employees, and their employee status usually took precedence over learning. This changed when students were given supernumerary status in the early 1990s, and a bursary of approximately half of their salary. However, the public services union, UNISON (2006), has been urging the government to scrap the bursary system for student nurses and pay them a 'decent wage' instead. The union's researchers found that 61 per cent of students were taking extra paid employment to supplement their income, and most of them acknowledged that this had a detrimental effect on their learning. Many students were in debt, 14 per cent of then owing more than £10,000. Two out of five students in the survey said they had seriously considered withdrawing from the course because they were having to take extra employment.

This movement has rumbled on since 2004, and on behalf of UNISON Harrison (2005) suggests that giving students more money can be achieved without ending students' supernumerary status. A report in *Nursing Standard* (Anon, 2006) indicated that a £10,000-a-year bursary was being recommended for nursing student.

In addition to Fretwell's research, a number of other studies were conducted during the 1980s to establish the factors that make clinical settings good or effective learning environments. One of these was Orton's (1981) study which concluded by identifying the characteristics of wards that showed High Student Orientation and those that reflected Low Student Orientation. In High Student Orientation wards respondents stated, for instance:

- 'All staff treated students with kindness and understanding and showed willingness to teach us.'
- 'Everyone got on well.'
- 'Each patient had individual total care however long it took.'
- 'Every nurse was made to feel important.'

On the other hand, in Low Student Orientation wards 96 per cent of students said they learnt more from other students than from qualified staff, and:

- 'The atmosphere was not very relaxed which made you worry about asking questions.'
- 'The ward sister did not respect us at all and gave us ten jobs to do at once.'

## Activity 4.3 – Creating a learning ethos in the clinical area

- Consider the findings and recommendations of the research studies just discussed.
- Do an itemised summary of your own identifying factors that make a good learning environment.
- How far does your own practice setting meet with the recommendations and the factors you've identified?
- Identify areas in which your practice setting is weak or could benefit from further improvement.

The responses to studies on clinical learning environments could be categorised as factors that promote learning in the clinical setting, and those that hinder, a number of which are identified in Box 4.2.

Box 4.2   Factors that promote learning and those that hinder learning in the clinical setting

*Factors that promote learning*

- Registrants' level of knowledge of their clinical specialism
- Adequate time to teach
- Practical demonstration of skills
- Students feeling they can take their time to practise the skills
- A learning ethos
- Teaching on a one-to-one basis
- Adequate staffing levels
- Adequate planning and preparation
- Supporting learning resources and information
- Approachable staff

*Factors that hinder learning*

- Interruptions
- Over-busy ward area
- Lack of time
- Attitudes of staff, patients and learners
- Standards of equipment
- Not enough information communicated
- Learner–staff ratio too high
- Inadequate staffing levels
- Student disinterested
- Disorganised programme of teaching
- Poor leadership

For non-hospital areas such as primary care settings, Gopee et al. (2004) make the following recommendations for enhancing them as learning environments:

- Mentor–mentee matching in accordance with seniority of practitioner and the student's particular learning needs.
- Management support to enable designated time to be given for mentoring, so that students and mentors feel time spent in this way is valued by their seniors.
- Raised awareness of the need to integrate theory and practice.
- Ensuring student practice outcomes are achievable, for example carrying out dressings might not be available in, say, placement with school nurses.
- Prior notices of placement and appropriate timing, for example not allocating student to school nursing placement during school holidays.
- Ongoing professional development for all grades of staff, for example in Professional Development Units.
- More effective communication at all levels and trust–university–mentor partnership.
- All mentors (and practice teachers) ensuring that they maintain the relevant NMC's standards.
- Access to clinical supervision for all qualified staff.

In more recent studies on clinical learning environments, Wood (2005), for example, reports on the experiences of a group of pre-registration mental health nursing students during practice placements, which indicated that they experience 'conflicting pressures', while their mentors experience difficulty supporting them because of high clinical workload.

Mikkelsen Kyrkjebø and Hage (2005) report on a Norwegian study examining nursing students' development of new knowledge in clinical practice and of health-care processes, cross-professional collaboration, and the handling of adverse events. The findings suggest a deficiency in improvement in knowledge in clinical practice and the existence of a theory–practice gap. The authors recommend a change in the culture within healthcare and health professional education to utilising learning models that encourage reflection, openness and scrutiny of underlying individual and organisational values and assumptions.

Henderson et al. (2006) report on an Australian study exploring students' percep-tions of psychosocial support available in clinical learning environments. They found that the medium for developing mentor–mentee relationships and students feeling part of the team were significant factors in enhancing student learning during prac-tice placements.

These more contemporary study findings related to mentors' workload, theory–practice gap, organisational values and psychosocial support reflect different issues to those identified earlier by Fretwell (1980) and Orton (1981). Based on the above accounts of the subject area, a clinical setting that consitutes a learning envi-ronment can be seen as one that comprises a psychosocial ethos and culture with related supportive resources that foster mutual learning amongst all stakeholder healthcare professionals, learners and clientele, and where care and treatment are founded on evidence-based practice. The recommendations from earlier and recent studies regarding aspects that constitute good and effective learning environments form key components of educational audits.

## Educational audit of practice placement settings

After Fretwell's and Orton's research, later studies on clinical learning environments (e.g. Rotem and Hart, 1995) focused more directly on exploring the factors that can be identified as criteria in educational audit tools to monitor the suitability of clini-cal settings for student placement. The criteria for suitability include evidence of a systematic approach to care delivery and holistic care (and the clinical setting's phil-osophy of care). Orton et al. (1993), for instance, specifically focused on educational auditing, and asked qualified staff and students the same questions separately, in relation to:

(a)  orientation to the placement;
(b)  theory and practice;
(c)  supernumerary status;
(d)  staff attitudes and behaviour;
(e)  the mentor;
(f)  progressive assessment.

Using questionnaires, under 'orientation to the placement' for instance, they asked qualified staff:

1. Do staff make students feel welcome on arrival?
2. Are students shown round the ward?
3. Are students allocated a mentor in their first week?
4. etc.

Correspondingly, they asked students:

1. Did staff make you feel welcome?
2. Were you shown round the ward?
3. Were you allocated a mentor in your first week?
4. etc.

Thus, having gathered data on the views of key players, Orton et al. (1993) then designed an education audit tool with specified standards for placement areas. It is an NMC requirement for annual educational audits of each clinical setting that is used for practice placement. Under the headings used by Orton and colleagues to explore the suitability of clinical settings as learning environments there are a number of 'ward learning climate indicators'.

## Optional activity – Strengths and weaknesses of your work base as a learning environment

The Orton et al. (1993) report contains the 'Ward Learning Climate Indicators' questionnaire used in the study. See if you can locate the publication from a university library and, if you can, then using the items in the qualified staff section, mark your own clinical setting in one of the four boxes for each item.

Alternatively, the actual items on the educational audit form used at your healthcare trust in partership with the university can be used similarly. A copy of the current completed audit form is usually lodged in the clinical setting. This exercise will highlight areas of strengths in, and where improvements can be made to, your own clinical setting as a learning environment. Can you do anything about the weaker points?

Each university devises its own educational audit tools in collaboration with the local trusts. The educational audit form titled 'Multi-professional Practice Environment Profile', which is constituted jointly by one university and the West Midlands South Strategic Health Authority (2006), comprises 40 standards criteria under:

1. Management of Practice Area;
2. Learning and Teaching Opportunities;
3. Assessment of Practice;
4. Effective Resources;
5. Quality and Evaluation of Practice.

Examples of standards criteria under 'Management of Practice Area', for instance, are:

- A philosophy of care is used that reflects core values of patient-centred planning and delivery of care.
- The provision of care reflects patient privacy, dignity, religious and cultural beliefs and practices.

Evidence needs to be available to demonstrate how each criterion is achieved. The educational audit document includes a section for recording the qualifications of each member of staff, of particular significance being which part of the professional register they are on and whether they have a mentoring qualification. Other post-registration qualifications are also recorded. Box 4.3 shows the content of another section of the audit form that contains key information that identifies the particular clinical setting.

---

**Box 4.3   Placement details**

**XXX  UNIVERSITY, NURSING, MIDWIFERY and HEALTHCARE**
**Multi-professional Practice Environment Profile**

Name of Trust/Organisation:
Site Location/Address:
Name of Ward/Department Unit/Organisation:
Telephone No:
Email Address:
Name of Placement Contact:
Type of Service Provision:
Date of Review:
Date of Previous Review:
Names of Reviewer/Review Team:
Name of Academic Link:
    Practice Educator:
    Practice Facilitator:
    Clinical Educator:
Name of Academic Institution/College Placing Students:
    University:
    College of Further Education:
    Other:
Work Patterns, e.g. length of shift patterns:
    am:
    pm:
    night:

---

Naturally, each item in this section of the audit form is important. The form also has a section for clinical staff to identify and list all the formal and informal teaching and learning opportunities that are available in the particular clinical setting.

## Activity 4.4 – Formal and informal learning opportunities

Identify and make two lists, one of all the formal learning opportunities that are available in your own clinical setting, and one of the informal ones. You might find it useful to discuss the activity with a colleague in the same clinical setting.

For formal learning, you might have mentioned lectures by the clinical nurse specialist for instance; and for informal learning opportunities you might have mentioned when the doctor changes a patient's medication. There are likely to be various teaching and learning opportunities in your workbase setting. Maybe one of the consultants holds regular formal teaching sessions for junior doctors, which all health professionals in the particular area are welcome to attend. Maybe pharmaceutical or medical devices company representatives give talks and demonstrations in the clinical setting. Further examples of teaching and learning opportunities that tend to be identified when completing educational audit forms are presented in Box 4.4.

If preferred, the resources for learning available in the clinical setting can be grouped as human and non-human resources. Formal learning opportunities, such as teaching sessions and skill demonstrations, require human resources and include inter-professional learning. Non-human resources include printed instructions on how to use equipment, learning about medications, ventilator monitors, or behaviour therapy. Many of the resources needed to deliver patient care can also be used for learning and for achieving clinical and managerial objectives. Other learning resources include a room that can be used for teaching and learning, with Internet-enabled computers, whiteboard, or flipcharts, for instance. The learning resource files compiled by clinical staff as part of projects or course assignments are also usually available for consultation and learning.

---

### Box 4.4 Formal and informal learning opportunities

*Formal teaching*

- Lectures by senior doctors
- Assessment-related teaching
- Interviews – initial, mid-placement and final
- Teaching while carrying out patient care (i.e. work-based learning)
- Setting students learning tasks
- Practice development manager's guidance
- Teaching by practice educator
- Cascade trainers
- In-service/post-graduate training
- Observing RNs, physiotherapists and other AHPs or doctors performing clinical skills

*Informal learning opportunities*

- Learning from patient with new condition
- Change in patient's condition discussed at handover
- Asking questions informally
- Reflection-in-action and reflection-on-action
- Informal chat in the staff room during coffee break
- Updating procedures and clinical guidelines folders and learning resources
- Access to computer databases

*Inter-professional learning*

As for inter-professional learning (IPL) in clinical settings, the concept is promoted in various authoritative documents (e.g. DoH, 1999, 2006a; ENB/DoH, 2001b; UKCC, 1999). Successful education programmes and projects (e.g. DoH, 2006a) are documented on the Internet and presented at conferences.

The basis for IPL is multi-professional working, in that to resolve the individual patient's or service user's health problem (or to avert it), a group of different health professionals such as nurses, doctors, dietitians, physiotherapists, and speech and language therapists input their own areas of professional expertise as appropriate. Multi-professional working can involve different health professionals attending to the patient, delivering their clinical input and withdrawing. These actions can be fragmented and inadequately co-ordinated and recorded. Inter-professional working implies better co-ordinated patient care with fuller communication, verbal and written, between different health professionals. Inter-professional learning extends the concept to the exchange of knowledge, understanding and clinical skills. Lloyd (1999) and Pirrie et al. (1998) also distinguish similarly between multi-disciplinary working and inter-disciplinary working.

IPL also comprises informal and formal learning. Informally, for instance, the nurse explains to the occupational therapist the plan of care for a particular patient and the rationales for each action. In turn, the occupational therapist designs a plan of actions and explains the rationales from their perspective. This could also form the basis for work-based learning, which is explored in detail shortly.

Formal IPL involves attending structured learning programmes, such as courses that are designed for specified health professionals, covering the physical, social and psychological basis for health and illness and the clinical skills that aid recovery. Some courses (or part of them) are designed for shared learning by, say, nursing and medical students (e.g. Freeth and Nicol, 1998; Morrison et al., 2004; Reeves and Pryce, 1998). Others, such as a course on counselling, might be designed for nurses, social workers and specific allied health professions.

Informal IPL refers to all modes of unstructured, incidental or opportunistic teaching and learning between different professional groups, while inter-professional education (IPE) refers specifically to university-designed courses that result in students being awarded diplomas or degrees. In their study of 'multi-professional education' (MPE), Pirrie et al. (1998: 415) use the term MPE to describe 'a range of situations in which students from different health and social care professions come together to enhance their understanding of particular elements of their professional practice'. They conclude that there are considerable benefits associated with MPE in healthcare, although it needs to be adequately resourced, and its success depends on the commitment of all staff involved.

Inter-professional education is defined by the Centre for Advancement of Interprofessional Education (1997: 1) as 'occasions when two or more professions learn from and about each other to improve collaboration and the quality of care' (see also Barr et al., 2005; Freeth et al., 2005). These definitions suggest that IPL is a more holistic term that encompasses all manner of inter-professional learning, while IPE refers specifically to learning by students on formal courses.

> ### Think Point 4.1 – IPL and IPE
>
> Consider to what extent IPL occurs in your work setting. In those settings where it does occur, is it linked to IPE?

Inter-professional learning has been explored for some time as either IPL, IPE or shared learning, by for example, Alaszwesski et al. (1998), Long et al. (2001), and Miller et al. (1999). A report by Hughes and Marsh (2006) for the *Creating an Inter-professional Workforce* programme presents a structure for implementing inter-professional working, which also identifies a number of themes and issues related to IPL.

In a study of post-qualified students undertaking an inter-professional studies programme, Salmon and Jones (2001: 18) found that skilful facilitation of learning was particularly important, and involved gaining an 'understanding of the knowledge bases, aspirations and values that underpin those (healthcare professions') roles'. Some of the issues related to IPL are as follows.

Hean et al. (2006) report on a study which concluded that different AHP students saw themselves as distinct from other professional groups. This is healthy as it enables them to establish their professional identity prior to exploring commonalties between them. However, when they identified the characteristics that made them different, for example physiotherapy students indicating that they believe that being a team player made them different, other groups also stated having this characteristic. This suggests that many of the characteristics of each AHP group are probably very similar. Naturally their areas of clinical expertise have different focuses. Reeves and Pryce (1998) found that medical, dental and nursing students revealed inconsistencies in their stereotypical attitudes towards the status of their intended professions. The authors suggest that these observations provide early evidence of key cultural, professional and institutional issues that need to be considered in planning and implementing inter-professional curricula.

Education programme planners need to be aware of the issues with IPE just highlighted so that they can make relevant adjustments to retain teaching effectiveness. However, healthcare learners benefit from inter-professional learning. One way that the care and treatment of particular patients are planned and delivered interprofessionally is through integrated care pathways. These in turn can form the basis for constituting learning pathways for students.

## Utilising learning pathways

The student's placement could in many settings beneficially incorporate patient journeys or patient care pathways identified by the Department of Health (e.g. 2002a, 2005, 2006b). Care maps, collaborative care pathways, multi-disciplinary pathways of care, are all terms that are used interchangeably. Once the care pathways for a particular patient has been formulated, it can be included in the student's learning pathway, which can be supplemented by pre-arranged lectures and workshops at the university, and by self-directed study.

In *Liberating the Talents,* the Department of Health (2002a) notes that 90 per cent of patient journeys begin and end in primary care. The Department of Health (2004b: 1) defines a patient pathway as 'the route that a patient will take from their first contact with a NHS member of staff (usually their GP), to the completion of their treatment. It also covers the period from entry into a hospital or a Treatment Centre, until the patient leaves.' The word *integrated* is added to care pathways to signify inter-disciplinary input.

The definitions of care pathways include that by Overill (1998: 93), who suggests that integrated care pathways provide 'locally agreed, multi-disciplinary practise-based guidelines and evidence where available, for a specific client group'. Care pathways specifically designed for particular illnesses are well documented in healthcare literature. Examples of this include van Wijngaarden et al. (2006) on thrombolysis in acute ischaemic stroke, McNicholl et al. (2006) on the care of dying patients, and Bowker et al. (2005) on the Type-1 diabetes mellitus. Several care pathways are also available on the Department of Health's website.

Research on care pathways includes an exploration of the application of Goldberg and Huxley's Pathway to Care by Issakidis and Andrews (2006) (in Australia), which revealed that being aged over 55 years or living in a rural area was associated with less access to certain healthcare sectors such as outpatient care. An evaluation of the application of the Liverpool Care Pathway for the dying patient indicates that the pathway made patient care clearer and uncomplicated, with specific methods of assessment and measurement of symptoms and outcomes (McNicholl et al., 2006).

A student on practice placement could encounter a patient whose journey through healthcare is taking them along the pathway identified in Figure 4.1.

The DoH (2006b: 1) identifies the patient pathway for a person referred for elective surgery through an 18-week journey from GP referral to the start of hospital treatment, although it indicates that most will be for shorter periods of time. The 18-week journey includes all the stages that lead up to treatment, including outpatient consultations and diagnostic tests and procedures. Integrated care pathways continue with the care and treatment required by the patient to the point of maximum recovery from the health problem.

The student can follow a patient's care pathway through the healthcare system closely to gain knowledge and understanding of the care and treatment required in particular illnesses. The student's learning pathway through the practice placement would involve exposure to, and engagement with, selected patient care pathways, supplemented in various ways, for example by practice-based teaching by the mentor and other health professionals.

HEIs work in collaboration with local trust clinicians to develop and implement learning pathway programmes in healthcare course curricula, based on patient journeys, with web-based scenarios for students to investigate. A suitable definition of learning pathways related to healthcare students' learning is difficult to locate. Essentially a learning pathway constitutes a selection of integrated care pathways for

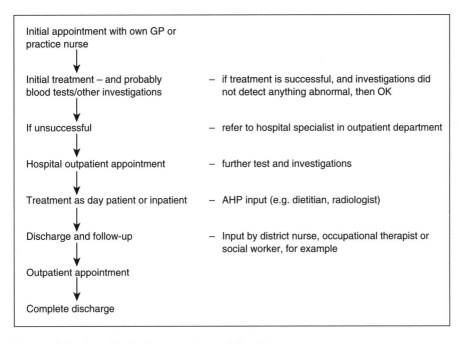

**Figure 4.1    A patient's journey through healthcare**

patients with different health problems that will enable the student to attain comprehensive learning about patient or service user care and treatment in the particular specialism, and achieve identified placement objectives. Furthermore, as care pathways incorporate involvement of an appropriate combination of nursing or midwifery, medical, social work and AHP staff, learning pathways are increasingly being referred to as 'inter-professional learning pathways'.

Pollard and Hibbert (2004) report on a project on enhancing student learning using patient pathways, and conclude that patient pathways constitute one way of turning students' learning during practice placements from an *ad hoc* set of activities into logical and organised experiences. Using patient pathways therefore offers a more structured approach to learning as opposed to relying on unplanned opportunistic, and therefore erratic, learning.

The learning pathway for a student on an Emergency Department placement could include the student starting with a day with the ambulance services, following a patient with a suspected fracture to the X-ray department, spending time working with plaster technicians, and so on. Furthermore, if the same patient also suffers from alcohol- or drug-related problems, for example, or displays aggressive or even violent behaviour, these themselves present instances for further learning for the student, the management of which can be explored up to maximum recovery.

Learning pathways have been identified as beneficial by Hutchings and Sanders (2001), for instance, who describe a successful project in which the development of learning pathways achieved its aims, which were to improve the quality of learning as well as being enjoyable, and promoting high-quality patient care. Students and clinical staff worked in partnership and had equal responsibilities for improving the quality of learning.

It is useful to note however that the notion of learning pathways is found in at least another two contexts. One of these is the arena of adult education in which individuals who have missed education opportunities during compulsory education years are enabled to learn through NVQ routes, and so on (e.g. McGivney, 2003). The notion of learning pathways also belongs to neuro-physiology when new learning can be identified along neuronal paths (e.g. Brown et al., 1999). However, this discussion indicates that integrated care pathways lend themselves to 'inter-professional learning pathways' by virtue of the range of healthcare professionals who might be involved in the patient's journey.

## Guidelines, policies and standards for practice placements

In *Helping Students Get the Best from Their Practice Placements* the Royal College of Nursing (RCN) (2002) specifies the responsibilities of various stakeholders, that is, those of the student, higher education institutions, service providers, personal tutors and mentors, for ensuring effective learning during placements. The responsibilities of the student encompass those before, during and after the placement. The student's responsibilities before the placement include:

- Reading the student handbooks related to the specific programme of study, including the assessment of practice that must be achieved.
- Recognising the purpose of the practice placement experience which is to learn nursing or midwifery care.
- Contacting the placement.
- Acting professionally with regard to punctuality and attitude, and dress according to uniform policy.

During the placement, the student's responsibility includes being proactive in seeking out learning experiences. After the placement, the student has a responsibility to take stock of their achievements, evaluate the placement itself, ensure all practice placement documentation is completed by due dates and reflect on the experience after completing the placement.

For mentors, the RCN publication states that good mentoring depends on well-planned learning opportunities and the provision of support and coaching for students. It lists and explains several actions that the mentor should take to fulfil their responsibility, which include:

- Contributing to a supportive learning environment and quality learning outcomes for students.
- Being approachable, supportive and aware of how students learn best.
- Having knowledge and information of the student's programme of study and practice assessment tools.

In a subsequent publication that constitutes guidance for mentors, the RCN (2005a) addresses how to mentor. This includes areas of accountability of mentors, helping students get the best from practice placements, including students with special needs, and support for mentors.

The underlying principles of the ENB/DH guidance document *Placements in Focus* (2001b) includes the need for a dynamic and proactive approach to the organisation, provision and assessment of practice experience. It indicates that HEIs and service providers have to think creatively about how to plan and provide practice placements that meet the needs of the new NHS, the wider healthcare sector and developments related to public health. Planning and provision should both take into account and value ideas and suggestions from students and draw on the experience and knowledge of other stakeholders. The guidance is intended to constitute a model of good practice. It focuses on four key aspects of practice placements, namely:

1. Providing practice placements.
2. Practice learning environment.
3. Student support.
4. Assessment of practice.

For the practice learning environment, the ENB/DH (2001b) indicates for instance that:

- The practice area should have a stated philosophy of care that is reflected in practice and in the curriculum aims.
- Care provision should be founded on relevant research- and evidence-based findings where available.
- Students should gain, where possible, experience as part of a multi-professional team.
- A learning resources area with relevant materials should be available for learning activities in the practice environment.
- Student feedback should be actively sought.

It also identifies how each component will be achieved by, for instance, placement providers, HEIs and students. Another authoritative body that provides guidelines on placement learning as a 'code of practice' for quality assurance is the Quality Assurance Agency (QAA) (2001). Mulholland et al. make further recommendations under the *Making Practice-based Learning Work* (2006) project.

## Work-Based Learning

In addition to statutory (e.g. DoH, 1999) and job-related reasons for the mentor function, other reasons and perspectives emanate from research findings and expert opinions. Kramer's (1974) research on newly qualified nurses constitutes one perspective that was mentioned in Chapter 1; another is the social learning theory advocated by Bandura (1977). Since this theory is firmly based on learning from other people, and this is how healthcare skills are usually learnt, the concept of work-based learning gradually evolved in recognition that learners learn knowledge and skills from competent professionals during care delivery. This section therefore examines what work-based learning (WBL, also referred to as practice-based learning) is, its features, research on the concept and related issues.

## What is work-based learning?

According to Guile and Young (1996), WBL is an innovative concept that firmly emphasises the importance of the workplace in competence development. They put forward a then relatively controversial idea that learning which does not take place in academic contexts was as important as learning within higher education, and the notion that all work-based learning is valid and creditworthy. Its value could there-fore be assessed on the basis of how far it is integrated, and possibly accredited within academic programmes, which Chalmers et al. (2001) and Hargreaves (1996) report as achievable. Credit rating of practice modules in the nursing curriculum is now commonplace.

Dewar and Walker (1999) suggest that WBL is primarily concerned with the process of learning and with encouraging the individual to be explicit about how and what they learn so that this experiential learning can also be assessed. Flanagan et al. (2000) note that WBL is the bringing together of self-knowledge, expertise at work and formal knowledge. It takes a structured and learner-managed approach to maximising opportunities for learning and professional development. Barr (2003) defined work-based learning as learning that takes place at work or learning that takes place away from work with the objective of improving performance at work. The definitions of WBL therefore emphasise the link between learning and work role, and interrelate:

1. Structured learning in the workplace.
2. On-the-job training opportunities.
3. Identifying relevant off-job learning situations.
4. Quantifying and credit-rating learning in practice settings.

Based on a project's findings, Foster (1996, cited in Flanagan et al., 2000) con-cludes that WBL comprises the following features:

- It is performance related, focusing on tasks arising in the workplace.
- It is problem based, focused on tackling complex work-based problems in the manage-ment of care.
- It is autonomously managed, with learners taking a large measure of responsibility for ensuring that they learn from their work activities.
- It is team based, tackling problems requiring effective co-operation between people with different roles and expertise.

### Issues and success stories related to WBL

Guile and Young (1996) suggest that one of the issues with WBL is the limitation of the concept of competence, which is what is learnt in WBL but which tends to incorporate behaviourist assumptions, with the tendency to relegate competency to reductionist descriptions of skill performance. They conclude that learning a competency should not be limited to 'know-how'; it should explicitly evidence the individual's understanding of the underpinning knowledge. The second issue involves comparability and equivalence between academic and work-based learning. As WBL is still a developing concept, a further, SWOT, analysis of the concept can be undertaken.

## Activity 4.5 – Critical analysis of WBL

Based on the above discussion, do a SWOT analysis of WBL and make notes on what you feel are the likely strengths, weaknesses, opportunities and threats related to WBL in your clinical setting.

In response to Activity 4.5, for strengths of WBL you might have mentioned 'learn hands-on clinical skills', for weaknesses 'lack of time to reflect', for opportunities 'the chance to learn specialist skills', and for threats you might have mentioned safety issues.

Following SWOT analysis, action can be taken to avoid or rectify weaknesses and threats. To resolve some of these dilemmas, Guile and Young (1996) recommend the use of the 'connective model', that is, the combination and inter-dependence of 'theoretical learning' and 'practical learning'. Theoretical learning provides concepts for analysing elements of practice, while practical learning constitutes workplace experience as a key source of competent development. Effective partnership between universities and healthcare providers is a necessary requirement for this to occur.

Components of a SWOT analysis of WBL are presented in Table 4.1, and you might wish to make notes on probable actions against each item.

Research studies and evaluation of WBL report variable findings. Some report how WBL programmes have been successfully implemented, while others highlight issues. For instance, Rattray et al. (2006) report on the evaluation of a critical care module that incorporated WBL and resulted in various benefits such as module credibility through its clinical focus. Waddington and Marsh (1998) explored work-based shared learning with a multi-grade, multi-skilled group of qualified nurses and healthcare assistants, and found that the perceived benefits included increased professional awareness of issues relating to standards and quality of care with enhanced communication and morale within the team.

On the other hand, Mallik and McGowan (2006) report on a multi-professional 'developmental project' on WBL which indicates that an inadequate supply of mentors results in inconsistency in the amount of mentoring students receive. Dewar and Walker (1999) report on an evaluation of WBL within a post-registration community health nursing degree programme which revealed a gap between the educational philosophy of WBL and the way in which it was delivered within the department concerned.

**Table 4.1  SWOT analysis of WBL and probable actions**

| SWOT analysis | Probable actions |
|---|---|
| *Strengths* <br> • Learn hands-on clinical skills <br> • Instils/builds confidence <br> • Involves multi-disciplinary team functioning <br> • Can visit other clinical areas <br> • Is grounded in the real world i.e. realistic within resource constraints <br> • Is more patient-centred <br> • Learners question rationales/effects of interventions <br> • Is dynamic, i.e. when the patient's condition changes, treatment is adapted | |
| *Weaknesses* <br> • Lack of time to reflect <br> • Work within resource constraints, therefore minimum/safe standards rather than optimum/expert <br> • Learner might not appreciate depth of theoretical knowledge required in e.g. blood pressure recording and monitoring <br> • In mental health, may not be able to get out of a patient interaction situation | |
| *Opportunities* <br> • Learn specialist skills <br> • To practise skills <br> • Explore if would like to work there <br> • Accredit practice-based learning with higher education credit points <br> • To develop clinical practice i.e. new ideas where there are problems, challenges <br> • Multi-professional learning <br> • Identify learning needs | |
| *Threats* <br> • Safety issues <br> • Relatives can oppose learners being involved <br> • Insufficient theoretical knowledge <br> • Reflection-in-action only, not reflection-on-action <br> • Less need for universities <br> • Big responsibility on the learner – they might not have the motivation or capacity to know what to learn and how | |

Rigorous quantitative studies are as yet in short supply, but Wilson et al. (1998) for instance report on a qualitative study of continuing professional development within a selection of healthcare organisations, which indicates that a number of inter-related factors contribute to WBL. These factors include: (a) the involvement of senior staff whose visions of learning make them role models for novice practitioners; (b) organisational structures and sufficient resources that support effective teamwork; (c) prompt feedback on performance to enable further learning to take place. The main conclusions indicate that the concept of a learning organisation was not readily recognised within healthcare, although some of their components were.

Ward and McCormack (2000) suggest that the development of a learning culture is becoming a dominant theme in the strategic plans of healthcare organisations. This is arising through a drive to improve standards of practice, bridging the perceived theory–practice gap and creating the means of integrating learning with practice. There have been many initiatives to create such a change, including CPD, reflective practice, clinical supervision and WBL.

Spouse (2001b) notes that successful WBL requires an organisational environment that supports learning through investment in staff, with staffing structures in organisations and trusts that free people up to work and learn collaboratively in a climate of trust, where investigations and speculations are fostered, and where time is protected for engaging in discussions about practice.

## Becoming a Learning Organisation

In line with Wilson et al.'s (1998) and Ward and McCormack's (2000) suggestions that organisational factors have a major influence on learning, gradually, the term *clinical learning environment* is being superseded by the concept of *learning organisation*. This concept is part of a trio of notions that include lifelong learning and learning society. It evolved with the development of various non-healthcare organisations such as banks, supermarkets, and so on, as learning organisations on the basis that they all learn from customer feedback and actively engage in ongoing staff training.

Watkins and Marsick (1992: 118) note that learning organisations are 'characterised by total employee involvement in a process of collaboratively initiated, collaboratively conducted, collectively accountable change direction towards shared values and principles'. The concept of a learning organisation is consistently becoming a feature of healthcare settings, and the ENB (1994: 11) noted that 'Because lifelong learning is not merely "keeping up to date" but is concerned with a flexible and enquiring approach to everyday events, the development of a culture of a learning organisation is an important part of the work of ... the NHS.' Hence the ENB suggested the creation of a culture of ongoing learning, and Watkins and Marsick suggest collective collaborative work and shared values as underpinning learning organisations.

The ENB (1994) viewed the development of an organisation that contributes to lifelong learning as consisting of eight key features. The idea of a learning organisation can, in future, be incorporated in educational audit tools for healthcare profession courses. Table 4.2 shows some examples of what each of the eight features includes.

## Issues Related to Practice Placements

One of the issues related to pre-registration nursing students is their supernumerary status accompanied by a relatively small bursary, as indicated at the end of Chapter 2. The latter is a reason for a number of students holding down part-time jobs. This, along with some students having a family to support, may result in their learning being compromised to some extent.

**Table 4.2   Implementing the key features of a 'learning organisation'**

| Characteristic | Brief details |
|---|---|
| The existence of a clearly articulated health policy which puts patients and clients at the centre | In ward/team philosophy/mission statement; include aspects of *Patients' Charter, Our Healthier Nation* |
| Effective communication throughout the organisation | Top-down and bottom-up communication; e-mails/memos, regular meetings |
| Key stakeholders and practitioners at all levels of the organisation are involved in its development | Multi/inter-disciplinary members involved; voluntary groups (e.g. Diabetes UK); doctors hold their own regular meetings |
| Staff development and performance review is in place for all practitioners | Development reviews, CPD strategy |
| Clinical supervision accessible for practitioners | For peer support; personal and professional development plans |
| Recognition that learning takes place in the workplace | Work-based learning; reflection-in/on-action; IPL |
| Determination guaranteed to translate rhetoric into action | For example, named nurse, team midwifery, standards |
| Commitment to encourage reflective practice | Making time for reflection-on-action |

One of the reasons for various guidelines on clinical placements being issued by the RCN, the QAA, the DoH (e.g. ENB/D.H, 2001b), and others at the turn of the century is the findings of research by Phillips et al. (2000), which documents various worrying weaknesses with prevailing mentoring processes. As noted in Chapter 1, this study highlights several issues or problems experienced by both mentors and students which resulted in redefinition of roles and change in educational preparation programmes for mentors.

Another reason is the increase in the number of students due to shortage of qualified nurses. This means more learners were to be mentored by fewer RNs. This also coincides with other research findings that some mentors were failing to fail students who were not competent, and that some newly qualified RNs were not 'fit for practice', that is, not clinically competent.

On the other hand, the heightened awareness of evidence-based practice means that students are more inquisitive about reasons for each step within clinical procedures. However, for various day-to-day reasons, some procedures are not performed exactly as the procedures manual states, and consequently the so-called theory and practice gap at times surfaces. From qualified healthcare professionals' and their managers' viewpoint these still constitute competent practice as procedures are adapted in accordance with resource availability and patient circumstances. For instance, if the moving and handling procedure or guidelines state that a hoist should be used to help a patient above a certain weight, but a hoist is not immediately available, then the RN could use alternative measures. The reason for this might not be immediately obvious to the student, and at times students refuse to participate in procedures that are not being performed precisely according to guidelines. They should be exploring how to adapt theories to practice instead.

## Chapter Summary

As with other components in this book, creating and maintaining an effective clinical learning environment is also identified as a key component of the mentor role. This chapter has focused on the different ways in which clinical settings can be effective as learning environments, and, having completed this chapter, you will have learned about:

- Students' perspectives on clinical placements such as their hopes and expectations, a ward orientation or induction programme, advanced preparation of learners and ensuring that course practice competencies are achieved.
- Research on clinical learning environments, which underpins the development of the tool for annual educational audits of clinical placement areas, learning resources (human and material) including inter-professional learning and learning pathways, and role models for learners in the clinical setting.
- The part played by national guidelines, standards and current policy documents on practice placements.
- What work-based learning is, how it is perceived and implemented, and an analysis of issues and success stories related to work-based learning, and successful implementation thereof.
- How learning can be enhanced for clinical settings to become learning organisations.
- Some of the main issues related to practice placements for students.

# FIVE

# Effective Practice and Clinical Practice Development

## Introduction

The key dimensions of being a mentor in healthcare professions incorporate practising one's craft to an extremely high standard. This in turn implies being conscious of the quality and effectiveness of one's practice, continuously ascertaining the evidence base of all clinical interventions and of the context in which care is delivered. Awareness of standards of practice involves being open minded with regards to novel methods of clinical interventions, of developments in one's own clinical specialism and in care and treatment in general. This chapter focuses on these dimensions of the mentor role, and covers:

- What effective practice is, and the mechanisms for ensuring and monitoring the effectiveness of care.
- Evidence- and research-based practice, what they are and how they can be achieved.
- Clinical practice development, what it is, why it is needed, and the management of such developments.
- The management of change, which includes the key components that are necessary for effective change implementation.

The NMC's (2006a: 54–5) standards document indicates, under the domain 'context of practice', that the mentor must 'support learning within a context of practice that reflects healthcare and educational policies, managing change to ensure that particular professional needs are met within a learning environment that also supports practice development'. Under 'evidence-based practice', the NMC indicates that the mentor must 'apply evidence-based practice to their own work and contribute to the further development of such knowledge, and practice evidence base'. The outcomes for these domains are:

1. *Context of practice*
   (a) contribute to the development of an environment in which effective practice is fostered, implemented, evaluated and disseminated;
   (b) set and maintain professional boundaries that are sufficiently flexible for providing inter-professional care;

    (c) initiate and respond to practice developments to ensure safe and effective care is achieved and an effective learning environment is maintained.

2. *Evidence-based practice*
    (a) identify and apply research- and evidence-based practice to own area of practice;
    (b) contribute to strategies to increase or review the evidence base used to support practice;
    (c) support students in applying an evidence base to their own practice.

## Chapter outcomes

On completion of this chapter you should be able to:

1. Explain why effective care and clinical practice development are key components of the mentor role.
2. Analyse the concepts of effective care and clinical practice development, and identify their inherent components.
3. Evaluate how mentors can engage in, develop and disseminate effective practice.
4. Ascertain and analyse what evidence-based practice is and how the mentor engages in this.
5. Critically evaluate the implementation of research findings, and the management of change.

## Effective Practice

Effective clinical practice is a concept that is closely related to quality assurance and is part of the agendas in the UK of clinical governance and the NHS Institute for Innovation and Improvement (NHS III) (2007) (previously the NHS Modernization Agency). Effective care (NMC, 2006a) is a concept that is an integral component of evidence-based practice and is closely related to the terms *clinical effectiveness* and *patient outcomes.*

    Clinical effectiveness refers to the extent to which specific clinical interventions, when deployed in the field for a particular patient or population, do what they are intended to do, that is, restore and improve health and secure the greatest possible health gain from the available resources (DoH, 1996). The RCN (1996) took this definition a stage further, indicating that clinical effectiveness is about applying the best available knowledge, which is derived from research, clinical expertise and patient preferences, to achieve optimum outcomes for patients. It emphasises maximum restoration of health, which is undertaken to the highest standard achievable. The three stages for achieving clinical effectiveness are (DoH, 1996):

- Obtaining evidence – from research published in journals, databases, clinical guidelines and so on.
- Implementing the evidence.
- Evaluating the impact of the changed practice and readjusting practice as necessary, usually through clinical audit and patient feedback.

The word *effective* is an adjective, which according to the dictionary (Brown, 2002: 794) means 'capable of producing results or a condition, and having the function of accomplishing or executing'. It can be used interchangeably with 'efficacious' and 'productive'. Related to the mentor role, the word effective therefore implies that the qualified healthcare professional accomplishes the goals in their patients' plans of care and treatment (or care pathways) as intended.

The three stages of achieving clinical effectiveness incorporate evidence-based practice and clinical practice development, which are examined in detail shortly. Achieving the goals of care and treatment also belongs to the arena of *patient outcomes*. This term has been explored for several years, and is defined according to the research it is connected with, as documented by the RCN (2004). However, despite the logic in ascertaining patient outcomes, there is a lack of consensus with regard to how patient outcomes are achieved, and therefore it remains in the background as an essential notion warranting further research and refinement.

Effective care, clinical effectiveness and practice development all aim to monitor and improve the standards and quality of healthcare delivery, which is also a function of the NHS III. The aim of the NHS III is:

> to support the NHS with high-impact solutions to some of its biggest challenges, as well as innovative ideas, new practices and technologies that will really make a difference to the delivery of patient care. The mission of the NHS Institute for Innovation and Improvement is to improve health outcomes and raise the quality of delivery in the NHS by accelerating the uptake of proven innovation and improvements in healthcare delivery models and processes, medical products and devices and healthcare leadership. (2007: 1)

The NHS III's (2007) priorities include work on '18-week wait' (DoH, 2006b), 'healthcare associated infections', and 'primary care and long term conditions'. The remainder of this chapter focuses on EBP and practice development, which are also components of clinical effectiveness.

## Evidence-based Practice (EBP)

One of the crucial components of effective practice and clinical governance is evidence-based practice, a concept that has been gradually adopted in all areas of healthcare. As indicated at the beginning of the chapter, besides being one of the NMC's (2006a) competences for mentors, EBP is also usually a component of the codes of practice of healthcare professionals. So what is EBP?

## What is evidence-based practice?

Evidence-based practice is closely associated with evidence-based medicine, and Doctor Archie Cochrane is renowned for being one of its principal initiators (Clarke, 1999). Sackett et al. (2000) are also well known for being advocates of EBP, and according to them EBP is the conscientious, explicit and judicious use of current best evidence in making decisions about the care of individual patients.

The key reasons for the adoption of EBP in healthcare is the move towards ensuring patient involvement in their care and treatment, the rise of consumerism and the shift from traditional or routine procedures to more objective scientific working (Dale, 2006).

Another term related to EBP is evidence-based healthcare (EBHC), and it has permeated various areas of healthcare in the form of evidence-based nursing, evidence-based management and evidence-based education. EBHC is defined by Gray (2001: 9) as 'a discipline centred upon evidence-based decision-making about groups of patients, or populations, which may be manifest as evidence-based policy-making, purchasing or management'. EBHC can be distinguished from EBP in that the former tends to refer to groups of patients, while the latter can refer to single clinical interventions. According to Gray there are five key elements of EBP, namely:

1. Decisions are based on best evidence.
2. The nature and source of evidence are determined by the problem.
3. Best evidence integrates research and personal experience.
4. Evidence is translated into action that affects patients/service users.
5. These actions are continually appraised.

 **Think Point 5.1 – Best evidence**

EBP therefore refers to the use of 'best evidence' and is based on national and international standards. How do we know that the way we provide care and treatment in our workplace is based on the 'best evidence' currently available?

Research evidence is available from national computer databases. However, Gray (2001) indicates that although the best evidence of effectiveness of particular clinical interventions comes from well-designed research, other evidence of best practice, referred to as 'best evidence available', needs to be considered seriously. There are several likely sources of best evidence of good practice, including:

- policy directives (from the Department of Health);
- specialist and research conferences;
- professional journal articles;
- overview of evidence on specific topics on computer databases;
- textbooks;
- suppliers' information;
- unpublished research;
- complaints from patients with a particular health problem;
- colleagues and peer contact – uni- or inter-disciplinary professionals;
- clinical guidelines;
- the patient/service user/their family;
- personal intuition;
- trial and error;
- personal experience.

## How is EBP achieved?

There are various ways in which EBP can be obtained. Healthcare professionals can search for evidence of the effect of particular clinical interventions and best evidence on computer databases such as the Cochrane library, MEDLINE or Cumulative Index to Nursing and Allied Health Literature (CINAHL), or they can do a manual search of literature.

There are various organisations that store and provide systematically reviewed (or critically appraised, or meta-analysed) research on different healthcare topics. The Cochrane systematic reviews library (available from http://www.cochrane.de/default. html), which stores research evidence that has been critically appraised or systematically reviewed, is one of them. Sleep and Clark (1999: 306–7) define a systematic review as 'a rigorous and exhaustive process for searching and appraising both published and unpublished literature on a specific aspect of healthcare … they adhere to strict scientific design in order to make them more comprehensive, to minimise the chance of bias, and so ensure their reliability'.

The strengths of the assembled research literature can be classified as a hierarchy of levels or grades of evidence, in order of validity and significance. For instance, Gray (2001) supports *Bandolier's* (a monthly journal on evidence-based practice) (1995) classification of the strengths of evidence, which is as follows:

- Type I:   Strong evidence from at least one systematic review of multiple well-designed randomised controlled trials (RCT).
- Type II:  Strong evidence from at least one well-designed RCT of appropriate size.
- Type III: Evidence from well-designed trials without randomisation, single group pre- and post-experiment cohort, time series or matched case-control studies.
- Type IV:  Evidence from well-designed non-experimental studies from more than one centre or research group.
- Type V:   Opinions of respected authorities based on clinical evidence, descriptive studies or reports of expert committees.

Alternatively, the strength of evidence is ranked as grades I, II, or III (McInnes et al., 1998):

- Grade I:   Generally consistent finding in a majority of multiple acceptable studies.
- Grade II:  Either based on a single acceptable study, or a weak or inconsistent finding in multiple acceptable studies.
- Grade III: Limited scientific evidence that does not meet all the criteria of acceptable studies or absence of directly applicable studies of good quality. This includes unpublished research reports and expert opinion.

Other organisations categorise evidence differently but they are essentially similar. Evans (2003) explored various such classifications and concluded that the appraisal of evidence should also include assessing the evidence's effectiveness, appropriateness and feasibility. Nonetheless, Sackett et al. (1996), Rolfe (1999) and others indicate strongly that RCTs must not be treated as 'gold standards'. Thompson (1998) and others indicate that EBP should take personal experience, intuition and patients' reports into account. The benefits of EBP are that healthcare professionals can (Kopp, 2001):

- Inform or advise patients more accurately.
- Make better use of limited resources.
- Instigate appropriate and up-to-date interventions.
- Measure practice against appropriate guidelines or standards.
- Provide a more informed decision-making process to previously untreatable or more expensive treatments.

However, there can be barriers to implementation of EBP. These barriers are similar to those that present as obstacles to implementation of research findings and are examined shortly. Kopp (2001) suggests that such barriers include a lack of awareness of evidence, and of self-confidence, peer support, or resources. Furthermore, Sackett et al. (1996: 71) suggest that 'practice risks becoming tyrannised by evidence … [but] without available evidence, practice risks becoming rapidly out of date to the detriment of patients'.

The difference between research-based practice and EBP is that research-based practice of clinical interventions allows consideration usually only of findings of quantitative research, while EBP also considers descriptive or qualitative studies, professional experiences, intuition (Benner, 2001) and tacit knowledge (when we know more than we can evidence or tell) (Polanyi, 1958).

The York University NHS Centre for Reviews and Dissemination is another resource centre for EBP. There is also the quarterly journal *Evidence-based Nursing*. The Health Technology Assessment programme (DoH, 2006c) is a government-funded venture that appraises research information, including costs and effectiveness, and is made available to NHS workers. A good resource for how to critically appraise research papers is Greenhalgh's book *How to Read a Paper* (1997). Typical headings for critical appraisal of a research study are:

- How clear and specific is the research question?
- Was the research funded by a particular organisation and, if so, does the researcher hold any allegiance to them?
- Is the research design the most appropriate to answer the research question?
- Are the sampling strategies the most appropriate?
- Precisely what was measured?
- Precise details of how the data was collected.
- How researcher effects and other intervening variables were controlled.
- Was the framework or method used for analysing the data the most appropriate?
- Are the statistical tests used appropriate and accurately documented?
- Are the conclusions drawn logically argued and is the generalisability statement justifiable?
- To what extent is the study relevant to clinical practice in the particular clinical setting?
- Does the dissemination of the study indicate frameworks for implementation, including resources required such as costs?

Much more detailed appraisal considerations are pretty well publicised, a good example of which is offered by McCaughan (1999). It is in the interest of the implementer of a particular component of EBP to examine closely and carefully the critical appraisal already conducted by established organisations, who in fact are also likely to have accessed and appraised the original study report.

## The mentor's role in identifying, disseminating and applying research findings

Identifying existing research on particular healthcare topic areas has become increasingly easier with wide availability of electronic databases such as the Cochrane library and MEDLINE. However, the actual dissemination of research findings is not as effectively achieved. Whether it is the findings of the healthcare professional's own research or those of studies encountered at conferences or on courses, the ultimate stages of research studies entail critiquing the study or studies, systematic dissemination and implementation of the findings.

The mentoring role includes awareness of research related to the mentor's own area of healthcare, and sharing such knowledge as appropriate, that is, dissemination. Scullion (2002) suggests that dissemination is a vital yet complex process that aims to ensure that key messages are conveyed to specific groups via a wide range of methods such that it results in some reaction, some impact or implementation. The key elements of dissemination strategies are the source, the message, the medium and the target users. Scullion suggests that effective dissemination can be achieved by:

- journal articles/editorials/short reports;
- feedback to research subjects;
- in-person support mechanisms;
- journal clubs, seminars;
- conference presentations;
- poster presentations;
- publishing as books/chapters;
- inclusion in curriculum;
- newsletters;
- designing educational materials.

However, McKenna (1995) notes that just getting the findings or a new idea published in a professional journal amounts to researchers simply reporting their findings, making recommendations and opting out, in the hope that someone will implement their recommendations. Scullion (2002) suggests that the main barriers to the dissemination process are: poor reading habits of nurses resulting in them being unaware of research findings, lack of time, lack of knowledge, negative attitudes towards research and information overload.

Furthermore, even with effective dissemination, there can be obstacles to implementation of research findings. Hunt (1981) identified the 'major obstacles to applying research in practice' as nurses not knowing about research findings, not understanding them, not believing in them, not knowing how to use them, and not being allowed to use them. Although Hunt's observations were published more than two decades ago, many of them still apply today. Hunt (1997) further indicates that other barriers to research implementation faced by nurse managers and clinicians include:

- Lack of critical appraisal and research skills.
- Lack of time to undertake research.
- Not having access to the right resources.
- An organisational and managerial ethos and culture expecting instant answers.
- Lack of power and financial control to make things happen.
- Lack of valid research on any one topic, or of user-friendly reviews and guidelines.

---

 **Thinking Point 5.2 – Barriers to implementing research findings**

Hunt's suggestions are at least a decade old. Consider how far these suggestions are still prevalent in the context of present-day healthcare settings, both in general and in your own practice setting.

---

McCaughan et al. (2002) explored acute care nurses' perceptions of barriers to using research information in clinical decision making, and identified them as:

- Problems in interpreting and using research, as it is seen as too complex, 'academic' and overly statistical.
- Nurses who feel confident with research-based information perceive a lack of organisational support.
- Researchers and findings lack clinical credibility and fail to offer sufficient clinical direction.
- Some nurses lack the skills and motivation to use research themselves.
- Participants like research messages passed on to them by a third party rather than becoming directly involved themselves.
- Rejection of research knowledge is not a barrier to its application, but the presentation and management of research knowledge in the workplace represent significant challenges for clinicians, policy makers and the research community.

## Activity 5.1 – Barriers to implementation of research findings

Re-read the barriers to implementation of research findings identified by Hunt and McCaughan in the previous bulleted lists, and consider what you see as barriers at your workplace, at ward or trust level, and make some notes.

Implementing changes to practice is examined later in this chapter. Palfreyman et al. (2003) explored nurses' and physiotherapists' sources of knowledge and perceived barriers to EBP, and found that although both parties access a wide variety of sources of knowledge, both professions have problems overcoming the barrier of time. Furthermore, nurses are more likely to use policy and procedure manuals, but rate themselves as having poor EBP skills. Hunt (1997), however, suggests that these issues can be resolved by:

- Making research available and accessible by development programmes.
- Providing research advice and support.
- Providing nurses with the appropriate skills.
- Changing attitudes.

On the other hand, Scullion (2002) notes that current commitment to research and EBP will have limited impact on patient care unless similar commitment to dissemination and implementation is established at both corporate and individual levels. Rycroft-Malone et al. (2002) note that successful implementation of evidence into practice is a function of three elements, namely the nature of the evidence, the context in which the change is to take place and the way the process is managed. They suggest a framework based on these elements for both implementation of novel practices and subsequent evaluation.

In the mentoring role, research-based practice is an inherent component, EBP can be a permanent feature, and 'where's the evidence?' sounds like a confrontational question. The healthcare trust's clinical procedure and guidelines, however, almost always include the evidence base for practice. Consider the following scenario which involves mentoring a student midwife.

## Case Study – Mentoring a student midwife

Sarah is the mentor to first-year student midwife, Helen. A 'triad'* assessment is being conducted with Helen by Sarah and Geraldine, the link tutor. The topic chosen is examination of the newborn.

Helen states that she is very nervous. She provides a full clinical picture of the woman and the baby in whose care she has been involved. Having confirmed the woman's consent, she then concentrates on the examination which she performs in a professional manner. There is however little communication with the mother. Helen has to be reminded of the need to complete the relevant documentation. Her hand is shaking as she writes.

Helen then produces and discusses an article regarding examinations of the healthy neonate. She needs some prompting when asked about the NMC's *Midwives Rules and Standards* and what she would do if she identified a deviation from the norm. When asked about her assessment of her performance, Helen is very self-critical, and feels that she did not do very well.

What are the key issues in this assessment situation? What are the ways in which the evidence base of Helen's performance influenced her performance, and what are the questions that Sarah and Geraldine might want to ask?

*triad* refers to a tri-partite assessment of competencies in the clinical setting that includes the assessee, their mentor and a midwife lecturer.

You do not have to be a midwife to ask relevant questions related to EBP and this case study. A number of issues surfaces when this scenario is put to a group discussion. In the context of the discussions in this chapter, all parties will question the strengths of the evidence that Helen seemed to have used during the procedure. They can be explored in the context of levels or grades of evidence available in relation to 'examination of the newborn'.

## Clinical Practice Development

Both concepts of clinical effectiveness and EBP imply changing the ways in which care and treatment are delivered if it benefits the patient or service user. Such changes are referred to as clinical practice development, which is the focus of the next section of this chapter. Clinical practice development is a key component of the NMC (2006a) competences for mentors. It explores what it is, the different reasons for clinical practice development, and how it can be managed. This is complemented by the next section which is on management of change.

### What is clinical practice development?

Clinical practice development implies changing the way particular clinical interventions are performed for the benefit of patients or service users. It has to do with improving and enhancing clinical practice where there is scope to do so. It refers to hands-on patient care interventions. Which developments in clinical practice are currently happening in your particular area of practice? What changes can be made or have been made recently to the specific care and treatments carried out in your clinical setting?

### Activity 5.2 – Clinical practice development

Reflect on how care is currently delivered in your workplace and explore whether any aspect of hands-on patient care has changed recently – in the last few months, or in the last year or two?

Next, identify an aspect of practice in your work setting that requires or could benefit from change, either in clinical care, patient teaching or organisation of care. State two examples of such potential changes.

So changes can be made in different components or dimensions of the healthcare professional's role. The mentor can influence the nature and direction of these changes. Examples of changes in hands-on clinical practice include:

- no-lift policy;
- use of patient-controlled analgesia;
- nurse-led specialist clinics;

- cognitive-behavioural therapy;
- nurse prescribing;
- using tympanic thermometers rather than glass thermometers;
- cardiac output studies in intensive care units;
- bedside handover.

Examples of changes in organisation or management of care include:

- introducing new shift system;
- integrated care pathways;
- team midwifery;
- outreach work;
- a quality assurance programme (e.g. patient satisfaction surveys);
- modern matron role in aspects of care (e.g. who does what to ensure hospital cleanliness);
- allowing parents to be present in the anaesthetic room;
- clinical supervision for peer support and CPD;
- a mechanism for reporting to colleagues from conferences and workshops.

Examples of changes in patient teaching include:

- health 'MOTs' conducted by practice nurses, SCPHNs;
- school nurses' advice to teenagers on sexual activity;
- teaching self-relaxation;
- teaching dietary control to a newly diagnosed diabetic;
- advising older people how to avoid hypothermia.

You could think of various instances of changes in teaching students and other learners, such as medical students, healthcare assistants, preceptees and inductees.

Practice development is defined by the RCN (2006: 1) as 'an approach that helps you, your team and organisation to provide care that patients feel is right for them'. This is a very brief definition. A more helpful definition is provided by McCormack et al., which states that:

> Practice development is a continuous process of improvement towards increased effectiveness in person-centred care, through the enabling of nurses and healthcare teams to transform the culture and context of care. It is enabled and supported by facilitators committed to a systematic, rigorous and continuous process of emancipatory change. (1999: 256)

According to Bryar and Griffiths (2003), practice development is taken to mean a broad range of innovations that are initiated to improve practice and the services in which that practice takes place. The term *innovation* differs from practice development in certain respects, especially in that the former refers to implementing something new and unprecedented. The dictionary (Brown, 2002: 1381) defines 'innovate' as introducing 'something for the first time, a new product, practice or method', and 'to make a change to something established'. Both activities refer to something developed necessarily in response to patient care needs, but development refers to a gradual progressive change and advancement. Innovation implies implementing a relatively radical new practice. The concept of change, however, can mean substituting something with something new, a development, or reverting to an older (but effective) practice.

Although nursing practice has been developing consistently over the years, one of the key stages in this is marked by the establishment of Nursing Development Units in the 1980s, which were clinical settings where appropriate changes in practice were implemented and empirically evaluated.

## Why clinical practice development?

One of the primary reasons that practice development is a mentoring role is that mentors are role models for their learners (Darling, 1984; NMC, 2006a). This reason complements the role or characteristic of the mentor as a standard-prodder, identified by Darling (1984), which implies that they should always be reflecting on whether their clinical interventions are of the highest standard known, with a view to making them even more effective.

The two NMC domains clearly indicate that the mentor must continually question the evidence base and effectiveness of the care they deliver. However, clinical practice is only one of the components of the RN's role that can be developed, others being their education and management roles. Another categorisation of healthcare professionals' roles, each of which can be further developed, is by the Department of Health (2004a) in the *NHS KSF*, which identifies all patient care activities under six 'core dimensions', namely: (i) communication; (ii) personal and people development; (iii) health, safety and security; (iv) service improvement; (v) quality; and (vi) equality and diversity. All categories imply quality assurance, but service improvement in particular relates to making 'changes in own practice and offer suggestions for improving services' (p. 70).

Practice development is evolving continually, and Collinson (2000) and Faugier (2005b) for instance take the concept further and discuss instances of the growth of 'nurse entrepreneurs'. The term *entrepreneur* of course refers to people who engage in novel, unprecedented ventures on a substantial scale, and implies being innovators. Liefer (2005) discusses government policy changes that allow entrepreneurial nurses to pave the way for nurse-led healthcare practices, for instance nurse-led leg ulcer clinics.

The RN's teaching role starts soon after registering as a nurse with the NMC, and they have to be qualified for one year before accessing the mentor preparation course. Therefore, although the mentor needs to monitor the evidence base and effectiveness of their practice, the extent to which they can engage in practice development is variable depending on experience and clinical circumstances. Becoming a nurse entrepreneur is an even longer-term prospect.

Government directives that encourage practice development include *Liberating the Talents* (DoH, 2002a), a document that encourages primary care nurses and midwives to develop their practice. It indicates that the Chief Nursing Officer's (DoH, 2002b) ten key roles for nurses provides a strategic framework for developing practice, and cites several examples of developments under 'setting up new services'. This is reinforced in various Department of Health documents, including *Modernising Nursing Careers: Setting the Direction* (DoH, 2006d) and ventures such as *NHS Innovations* (DoH, 2006e).

Practice development is also propelled by RNs' expanded roles. Previously known as extended roles, expanded roles refer to those clinical interventions that healthcare professionals engage in following relevant post-registration training and assessment.

With the implementation of the *European Working Time Directive* (DoH, 2004c) leading to reduction in doctors' working hours, an increasing range of clinical interventions that were previously doctors' roles are now also performed by other healthcare professionals. These roles afford healthcare professionals greater autonomy and further scope for decision making, and therefore creativity and consequent practice development, as also noted by the RCN (2005b).

A major study by the UKCC (2000) on expanded roles revealed that their impact on practice include:

- Continuity of care being regarded as the most important benefit.
- Practitioners being involved with work in care settings where there is a good skill mix, regular opportunities for CPD, and excellent communications and mutual respect within the healthcare team.
- Professional experience, motivation and use of intuition as well as education and supervision being important practitioners' abilities.

The study also concluded that to support role development, healthcare organisations must provide:

- Adequate training (i.e. CPD).
- Structures which support CPD.
- Management support, sustained by education and training.
- Change that is patient-led rather than management-driven.
- Clear guidelines and protocols.

## Management of clinical practice developments

### Concept analysis of practice development

Garbett and McCormack (2002) undertook a concept analysis of practice development based on an analysis of literature, focus group interviews with practice developers and telephone interviews with practitioners. A conceptual framework derived from the study comprises the purposes, attributes and outcomes of practice development (see Box 5.1).

---

### Box 5.1 Purposes, attributes and outcomes of practice development

The purposes of practice development are to:

- Increase the effectiveness of patient care
- Transform care and the cultures and context within which it takes place

The attributes of practice development are that it:

- Requires a systematic and rigorous approach
- Is a continuous process
- Is founded on various types of facilitation

---

*(Continued)*

The consequences of practice development include:

- For users – improved experiences of care in terms of their sensitivity to the needs of individuals and populations
- For practitioners – increased capacity for thinking creatively and more broadly
- Greater awareness of the impact of organisations on practice

---

Unsworth's (2000) concept analysis of practice development identified wide variations in the way the term is used, and resulted in a tentative list of critical attributes of practice development, which are:

- New ways of working which lead to a direct measurable improvement in the care of or service to the client.
- Changes which occur as a response to a specific client need or problem.
- Changes which lead to the development of effective services.
- The maintenance or expansion of business/work.

Titchen (2003) identifies three overarching themes that form the basis for effective practice development, which she refers to as the practice development diamond. The themes are (a) changing the practice philosophy; (b) the process of change in practice; and (c) investing in professional development. Page (2001) presents a framework of practice development using the Donabedian model, which incorporates developments instigated at individual level, team level, organisational level or at supra-organisational level (see Table 5.1).

The framework is comprehensive and, when all details are completed, it can also be used for ongoing and summative evaluation of the development after it has been implemented.

**Table 5.1   A framework for practice development**

| Practice development | Structure/approach | Process/deployment | Outcome/results |
|---|---|---|---|
| | Individual Performance Review/PD framework | Development of PD practitioner or each team member | Active participants Reflective practitioner |
| Individual | – | – | – |
| Unit/Team | – | – | – |
| Organisational | – | – | – |
| Supra-organisational | – | – | – |

*Source*: adapted from Page (2001).

### Activity 5.3 – Developing practice

Based on the list of developments generated as a result of Activity 5.2, think of two aspects of practice in your work base that could be developed. Consider and make notes on how the framework presented by Page (2001) can be utilised to change these two aspects of practice.

The practice development framework suggested by Page should enable you to take these developments further systematically if you so wish, and maybe within the context of management of change (discussed next in this chapter). The RCN (2006) also has a designated Practice Development Team that provides structured help, advice and support in various ways.

The resources that can help healthcare professionals include the journal *Practice Development in Healthcare*, and national conferences specifically on practice development. Several NHS trusts employ Practice Development Nurses or Facilitators. Some have Practice Development Units that conduct experiments on new modes of practice.

## Managing Change

All healthcare professionals will have encountered changes in the way care and treatment is organized and delivered in various clinical settings. It is therefore almost inevitable that mentors will be involved and participants in change, and they are expected to initiate it when appropriate. Therefore, the mentor needs to have knowledge and competence in managing change. It is important to distinguish between the concept of managing change from that of introducing or imposing change; the latter can be effected at short notice, but managing the change implies longer-term, planned, systematic and sustained activities. Change is ongoing in healthcare delivery but why do we have changes in healthcare in the first place?

### Why changes in healthcare?

### Activity 5.4 – Changes in healthcare delivery

Consider the points made about practice development earlier in this chapter, and think of as many reasons as you can for the continuing changes that occur in healthcare at ward level, hospital level and in primary care settings. Make notes on what the reasons for these changes are?

Chances are you will have thought of quite a few reasons for changes that you have observed in healthcare. They include government policy directives (such as *Agenda for Change*; DoH, 2001a), the need to improve practice, and learning from 'near misses', or mistakes. These reasons can be grouped under seven areas, as noted in Box 5.2.

---

### Box 5.2  Reasons for changes in healthcare

- *Change in medical technology* — New medical devices and equipment; use of computer networks and easier access to information

- *New knowledge* — Research and audit findings; expert guidelines

- *Safer and more effective products* — Consumable materials and hardware being superseded by more efficient ones

- *The nature of the workforce* — Workers of different age groups, and with domestic responsibilities; changes in qualified:unqualified staff ratio (e.g. healthcare assistants with different skills)

- *Revised policies and strategies* — Use of devices and strategies to prevent injury to staff, or to avoid 'hospital-acquired infections'

- *Quality-conscious consumers* — Consumer satisfaction surveys indicating the changes that should be made

- *Funding and budgets* — Availability and distribution of scarce resources

---

Mullins (2005) notes that change is an inescapable feature of both organisational and personal life. The sources of change can be grouped under those that are internal to the organisation and those that are external, as noted in Box 5.3.

---

### Box 5.3  External and internal forces of change

*External forces of change*

- Market forces (i.e. competition between similar organisations)
- Legislation (e.g. equal opportunities)
- Tax structures (e.g. changes in value added tax)
- New technologies (e.g. equipment, computers)
- Political – changes made to influence opinions

*Internal forces of change*

- Profitability (e.g. improved production facilities)
- Reorganisation – due to increase or decrease in demand for particular products
- Conflict between departments or people
- Changes in culture/social environment

*Source:* Mullins (2005).

However, some reasons can be both internal and external. For instance, if the quality of care is unsatisfactory, then the employees of the organisation will be aware of this, and they'll endeavour to rectify it, but the same issue might have been identified through external sources such as Healthcare Commission audits.

Five essential and inter-related factors that are crucial to the accomplishment of change were identified by the ENB (1987), suggesting that the change could succeed or fail depending on the effectiveness of each of the five factors in the chain. One weak link and the process of change could break down. The five factors are:

1. The innovation itself
2. The environment
3. The users
4. Change agents
5. Change strategies.

## The innovation itself

There are seven attributes that are necessary in the innovation or change if it is to be implemented successfully. These are:

- *Relative advantage* – the change must show that it has relative advantage over the status quo.
- *Compatibility* – the proposed change must be compatible with existing beliefs and values of the group at philosophical as well as pragmatic levels.
- *Communicability* – the ease with which the change can be understood.
- *Simplicity* – the ease or difficulty in the use of an innovation.
- *Trialability* – possibility of piloting the innovation.
- *Observability* – the change must be observable.
- *Relevance* – the degree to which the change is relevant for the particular clinical setting.

For example, if integrated care pathways (discussed in Chapter 4) are to be implemented, then does this system achieve these seven attributes? The specific meaning of the term innovation was explored earlier in this chapter under clinical practice development.

## The environment where change will be implemented

The second essential factor for effective implementation of change is whether the particular clinical setting is suitable and 'ripe for change'. It might not be 'ripe for change' if there is extensive resistance to change by the employees or team where change is to be implemented. An unsuitable time would be when there are too many unresolved issues or too many unfilled vacancies. There could also be barriers to change, which implies that organisational factors such as funding levels, politics or management are likely to obstruct change.

## The users

Another essential factor to consider in effective change implementation is the 'users' of the change. Rogers and Shoemaker (1971) identified six categories of users who are likely to be found in an organisation when change is envisaged. They are:

- *Innovators* – individuals who feel excited by novel practices that appear more effective and efficient.
- *Early adopters* – those who accept the change quite soon.
- *Early majority* – the first group to follow the early adopters.
- *Later majority* – other groups join the adopters of the change.
- *Laggards* – individuals who tend to lag behind.

Other individuals can be categorised as *rejecters*, that is, individuals who usually reject any change.

---

:💡: **Think Point 5.3 – Innovators, laggards and rejecters**

What, if anything, can clinical managers do about each group of staff identified in Rogers and Shoemaker's (1971) categorisation?

---

Healthcare managers can react or proact in specific ways towards each group of staff for managing the particular change effectively. For instance with:

- *Innovators* – use the energy, allocate responsibilities.
- *Early adopters* – recognise their motivation.
- *Early majority* – give sustained time and support.
- *Later majority* – reinforce by recognition and showing keen interest.
- *Laggards* – give extra support, prevent disillusionment.
- *Rejectors* – line manager to explore, as the individual might have evidence to the contrary, or might, for instance, be experiencing transient personal problems.

## Change agents

The change agent is the person who is appointed to advocate, implement or lead the change. He or she has five fundamental functions:

- To have thorough knowledge of the change envisaged.
- To identify the exact goals of the change.
- To develop strategies for introducing the change.
- To disseminate knowledge and strategies to relevant individuals and groups.
- To establish and maintain a working relationship with change users.

Sullivan and Decker (2005) indicate that some of the characteristics that successful change agents (or project managers) should cultivate and master are:

- The ability to combine ideas from unconnected sources.
- The ability to energise others.
- Have well-developed interpersonal and human relations skills.
- Integrative thinking: retaining big picture focus while dealing with specifics.

- Flexible, persistent.
- Realistic thinking.
- The ability to handle resistance.

**Table 5.2   Transactional and transformational leadership**

| Transactional | Transformational |
|---|---|
| • Is task centred | • Empowers relevant others |
| • Has a short/medium-term focus | • Inspires by vision |
| • Coaches and exercises sheltered learning | • Has a long-term focus |
| • Rewards formally | • Challenges |
| • Is comfortable, orderly | • Sees home and work lives as a continuum |
| • Separates home and work | • Rewards informally, personally |
| | • Is emotional and passionate |
| | • Simplifies and clarifies |

Change agents have to demonstrate leadership abilities, and the transformational leadership style is particularly relevant for managing change. Some of the key facets of this style compared to those of the frequently demonstrated transactional style are presented in Table 5.2.

Transactional leadership involves the orderly breaking down of tasks but this often leads to loss of vision and energy. On the other hand, transformational leaders keep a distance, take a strategic or 'helicopter' view of the whole picture, lead by being passionate about the task in hand, and empower.

## Change strategies

Strategies for change can be derived from existing models of change incorporating planned and systematic actions, based on underpinning beliefs and philosophies. There is a range of strategies that the mentor can choose from to implement change. One of the first steps in this venture is to do a SWOT or a forcefield analysis. SWOT analyses were introduced in Chapter 4, and an example of a forcefield analysis is presented in Table 5.3.

**Table 5.3   Forcefield analysis – named nurse**

| Driving forces | Restraining forces |
|---|---|
| • Government patients' charter | • Could feel threatened |
| • Patient choice – recognise dealing with care | • Patient may not like the nurse |
| • Sense of responsibility | • Shifts – practicality |
| • Direction for nurses | • Time factor |
| • Follow-up care – admission to discharge | • Staff disappointment, frustration |
| | • Patients/relatives frustrated/antagonised if nurse off duty |
| | • Dissemination of information (e.g. at ward rounds) |

## Activity 5.5 – How is change managed?

Consider, maybe in a small group of healthcare professionals working in different specialisms, any one of the changes identified in response to Activity 5.1, for example self-rostering or integrated care pathways, one that approximates a real change issue in the practice area of one of the group members. With the chosen change, do a SWOT or forcefield analysis in relation to your own clinical practice.

A number of strategies for change are available to the healthcare professionals to choose from, the most noteworthy of which are:

(a) Lewin's three-stage process;
(b) empirical-rational strategy;
(c) power-coercive strategy;
(d) normative-re-educative strategy;
(e) combined strategy.

Each of these strategies is based on different assumptions held by the change agent about the people who have to accept the change. The appropriate strategies vary according to different situations, and a combination of strategies can be used. The SWOT or forcefield analysis of the change topic that you have just performed can be part of the first stage of Lewin's (1951) change strategy. The analysis unfreezes the new concept.

### (a)   Lewin's three-stage change strategy

Lewin's three-stage process of change involves unfreezing the situation, implementing the change, and then refreezing it. This is obviously an extremely simplistic explanation of activities that warrant careful planning and conduct. Unfreezing can be achieved by the SWOT or forcefield analyses just discussed. The implementation of the change is referred to as movement, and refreezing refers to sustaining the change.

Following a SWOT or forcefield analysis, the actions that can be taken entail reducing the weaknesses and strengthening the driving forces. A format like the ones presented in Table 5.4 for introducing flexible hours, and Box 5.4 for peri-operative visiting can be utilised for this.

**Table 5.4   Forcefield analysis – introducing flexible hours**

| Probable actions | Driving forces | Restraining forces | Probable actions |
|:---:|---|---|:---:|
| ← | What people want | Long-term staff against | → |
| ← | Retention issues | Fear of coming off worse | → |
| ← | Encourage recruitment | 'Unfair' | → |
| ← | Staff morale | Fitting in with practical routine | → |
| ← | Maximum use of staff time | Not feeling part of the team | → |
| | | Staff morale | → |
| | | Lack of communication | → |

---

**Box 5.4    SWOT analysis – peri-operative visiting**

SWOT analysis                                                    Probable actions

**Strengths**
- Reduce anxiety
- Patient compliance up
- Post-operative compliance down
- Patient preference to nursing staff
- More interdisciplinary collaboration
- Patient divulges more information
- Continuity of care

**Weaknesses**

- Resources
- Time
- Maybe lack of knowledge
- Too many people disseminating information

**Opportunities**

- Role expansion
- Specialist role
- Education
- Increase cost effectiveness through patient compliance
- Enhance patient care

**Threats**

- Lack of continuity of care
- Cost – funding
- Patient information overload
- Elitism – conflict

---

*(b)   Empirical-rational strategy*

The empirical-rational strategy is used by the change agent by enabling the prospective users of the change to appreciate research findings or other evidence that indicates the need for change. It builds on the assumption that people are essentially rational, are guided by reason, and that if they can be helped to understand the reasons and processes of the proposed change, they are more likely to adopt it. Therefore this strategy is also based on empowerment through giving knowledge. Government health warnings are often based on this strategy.

*(c)   Power-coercive strategy*

Another strategy for implementing change is the power-coercive strategy, in which the change agent emphasises their position power by underlining political and economic dynamics to achieve the desired outcomes and, where necessary, the use of moral power, playing on feelings of guilt and shame. Coercion refers to very strong persuasion to accept the change and may incorporate potential threats and sanctions.

The assumption is that those in control of the organisation will identify the need for change, and people with less power will comply with their plans: If an empirical-rational approach does not work then a power-coercive strategy may be used but this does not usually prove as productive in the long term.

*(d)   Normative-re-educative strategy*
Some change topics necessitate predominantly a re-educative approach in that if the users of the change are unfamiliar with the novel idea, then acquisition of new knowledge and skills will be a prerequisite for the change. This approach is also based on the belief that individuals and groups are inherently seeking and accepting novel ways of practising their trade based on evidence or research.

---

 **Think Point 5.4 – Strategy for change**

It is likely that during your early years as a newly qualified health professional you were involved in some component of change. This encounter may have been deliberate or incidental. The change may have been initiated through internal or external forces. In relation to this, consider how:

1.   You reacted to the change.
2.   You as an individual (or within a group) accepted or resisted the change.
3.   Did you perceive any specific strategy used to bring about the change (e.g. power-coercive, empirical-rational, or normative-re-educative)?

---

Change has to come from within the organisation, that is, a bottom-up approach including active involvement in planning, implementation and evaluation of the process of change for successful implementation. These lead to increase in motivation and personal growth, alongside commitment and co-operation.

*(e)   Combined strategy*
An appropriate combination of the above four strategies may be structured to suit the innovation, the environment, the users and the change agent.

The concepts of practice development and change and innovations are widely discussed at national levels mainly at conferences and through benchmarking. Binnie and Titchen (1999) refer to these activities as a series of journeys, implying that awareness of new ways of working and change management are naturally evolving dimensions within healthcare professions. They also identify a number of principles for practice development, which include components such as promoting and supporting a climate in which work is experienced as intellectually stimulating, growth is fostered, and the relevant infrastructure is well developed.

## Chapter Summary

This chapter has focused on the mentor's role in effective practice and clinical practice development. Having completed this chapter you will have learned about:

- What effective practice and clinical effectiveness are, and their relevance for the mentor role.
- Evidence-based practice, addressing what it is and how it is achieved; research-based practice; and the mentor's role in identifying, evaluating, disseminating and applying research findings, and how to overcome barriers to implementation.
- Clinical practice development, what the term means, including a concept analysis of practice development, the reasons for developing practice and how they can be managed effectively.
- Managing change, incorporating the key reasons for constant changes in healthcare, and the components necessary for effective change implementation, namely the nature of innovations, clinical environment factors where change is to be implemented, the users of the change, change agent(s) and change strategies.

# SIX

# Assessing the Learner's Knowledge and Competence

## Introduction

One of the most fundamental functions of the mentor is to assess learners' clinical knowledge and competence. This chapter focuses on this, and covers:

- What the term *assessment* means in the context of assessment of healthcare profession students' clinical competences.
- Why we need to assess our students and learners.
- Who assesses learners' competencies, other than their mentors?
- How assessments are conducted, including various principles and strategies.
- Implementing policies and approved assessment procedures in assessment of professional practice.

Assessment of professional knowledge and competence is therefore an integral part of all healthcare courses. One of the principal purposes of mentoring courses is to equip course attendees with the capability to assess learners' competencies, and at the end of each assessment the mentor makes a decision about whether the learner is competent to perform each of these skills independently, unsupervised and safely, and signs the learner's competencies booklet accordingly. There are a number of factors that the mentor needs to take into consideration to fulfil their assessment function effectively. These factors are explored in this chapter from the perspectives of what assessments are, why we perform them, when, who performs them, and the range of methods available. These points essentially constitute the principles and processes of assessments. Problems with assessments, as well as past and present criticisms and how they can be averted or resolved, are addressed in Chapter 7.

In its specification of competence and outcomes for the mentor under 'Assessment and accountability', the NMC (2006a: 50) indicates that the mentor should be competent to 'assess learning in order to make judgements related to the NMC standards of proficiency for entry to the register or for recording [registering] a qualification at a level above initial registration'. The outcomes of this particular mentor competence are:

- Foster professional growth, personal development and accountability through support of students in practice.
- Demonstrate a breadth of understanding of assessment strategies and ability to contribute to the total assessment process as part of the teaching team.
- Provide constructive feedback to students and assist them in identifying future learning needs and actions, manage failing students so that they may enhance their performance and capability for safe and effective practice or be able to understand their failure and the implications of this for their future.
- Be accountable for confirming that students have met the NMC or not met the NMC competencies in practice, and as a sign-off mentor confirm that students have met or not met the NMC standards of proficiency and are capable of safe and effective practice.

The concepts that are inherent to the principles of assessment implicated in the aforementioned NMC outcomes are therefore essential.

## Chapter outcomes

On completion of this chapter you should be able to:

1. Identify what assessments are and precisely on which specific elements of healthcare courses students are assessed.
2. Enunciate a number of reasons for assessment of clinical skills and knowledge of students on healthcare profession courses.
3. Identify who assesses, including the roles of self- and peer assessment.
4. Explain a range of ways in which student assessments are conducted, and the various key principles of assessments that need to be adhered to by the assessor.
5. Explain the processes of the management of assessment of clinical competencies, and how assessments can meet essential criteria such as validity and reliability.

## What are Assessments?

To begin to examine the principles and processes of assessments, it is useful to establish first what you as the healthcare professional already know about assessments of competencies.

## Activity 6.1 – What do you already know about assessments?

1. Think of the courses you have already attended, and any one(s) you might currently be on. Think also of your contact with learners and students on various programmes of study. What are the various methods of assessments that are used to assess your and other learners' knowledge and skills? Jot down as many methods as you can think of.

2. Consider what else you already know about assessments, which aspects of assessments you are unclear about, and what else you feel you need to know about assessments. Make written notes of your responses.

So what do you already know about assessments? In response to Activity 6.1, you may have thought that assessment of clinical skills is best carried out by direct observation of the learner's performance, and by reflective practice write-ups. Essays and written examinations are used for the assessment of theory. Most of these will be examined in this chapter under 'how to assess'.

Examples of assessments of theory and practice in healthcare education programmes include:

- structured essays;
- objective or multiple-choice tests;
- profiles and portfolio write-ups;
- practice-based competencies;
- care or case studies;
- seminars;
- written examination;
- OSCE (i.e. Objective Simulated Clinical Examination);
- short-answer questions;
- practical assessments in skills laboratories;
- individually negotiated projects;
- longitudinal studies.

Your response to what else you feel you need to know about assessments obviously depends very much on your experience, existing knowledge and understanding of the concept, and it varies between individuals. You might have felt for instance that you could do with knowing more about formative, summative, continuous, peer/ self-assessment, or about practice competencies.

## What do we mean by assessments?

A number of assessment methods such as written examinations, practical assessments and projects have just been identified.

### Activity 6.2 – Assessments I've passed

To explore this area further, first look back to a course you attended, preferably recently, and make notes on the following:

- A list of assessments that you had to pass to complete the course successfully.
- When exactly during the course were you assessed?
- Specifically what was assessed?

If you were assessed by continuous assessment, then you would have been exposed to a range of assessment components on different occasions, during both clinical placements and in university skill laboratories and classrooms.

### Definitions of assessment

The dictionary (Brown, 2002: 331) states that the word 'assess' originates from the Latin word '*assidere*', which means sit by or beside, which implies a close relationship and sharing an experience. The word also means 'estimate the extent, value or worth' of something. Therefore, assessment tends to imply staying by the learner's side and observing them perform a clinical skill with a view to stating at the end of the performance whether the skill was carried out competently. It also seems to imply being supportive and identifying subsequent learning needs.

Taking a step back, however, it is important to note that an assessment is not an activity we perform only occasionally to fulfil our work role. We assess life situations all the time before we take any action, whether it is to do with assessing whether to wear a coat when going out, based on the perceived weather and temperature outside, whether it is safe to overtake when driving, or whether we can treat ourselves to a delicious cake while bearing in mind the day's calorie intake. Such assessments do not result in someone awarding us a pass or fail but they still involve assessing stimuli or data prior to making decisions.

Assessment is also reflected in patient assessment, which entails collecting information and identifying actual and potential patient problems from the data, from which a plan of care is constituted. Student assessment, however, is related to collecting information as evidence of the student's ability to perform particular clinical skills or competencies. Some of the core skills necessary for assessing patients' needs and problems are also relevant for assessing learners. These are observing, measuring and interviewing (Open University, 1984). These skills also apply to assessment of students' knowledge and skills. For assessing health profession learners' clinical competencies and related knowledge, assessment can be defined as the purposeful observation and questioning undertaken to ascertain the learner's ability to perform particular clinical interventions in precise accordance with established or approved guidelines, and their knowledge of rationales for each action. As Curzon (2001) suggests, assessments involve collecting, measuring and interpreting information related to students' responses to the process of instruction.

Other definitions are provided by Nicklin and Kenworthy (2000) for instance, who define assessment as a measurement that directly relates to the quality and quantity of learning and is therefore concerned with students' progress and attainment. While quantity of learning could imply the number of skills or part skills that the learner has already learnt, quality of learning refers to how thoroughly the skills have been learnt. The latter would also suggest progress and identifying areas of further learning.

## What do we assess?

The NMC's *Standards of Proficiency for Pre-registration Nursing Education* (2004b) identify the exact competencies and outcomes that each student needs to achieve to gain entry to the NMC register, as does the HPC for AHP students. There are also 'specialist practitioner outcomes' for SCPHNs (NMC, 2004d) for instance, as there are criteria, competence and outcomes for mentors and practice teachers (NMC, 2006a). These factors or features are reflected in the course and modules' aims and learning outcomes, in theory and in practice components.

The UKCC (1999) advocated an outcomes-based competency approach to education which encourages the development of knowledge, understanding, practical and technical skills, attitudes and values. The NMC (2005d) has retained this approach and identifies competence as relating to the need for the student to demonstrate their 'capability' in certain skill areas to a required standard at a point in time, and that competencies are component skills which contribute to being competent and achieving the standards of proficiency for registration. A widely accepted definition of competence is that the term is used to describe the skills and ability to practise safely and effectively without the need for direct supervision (UKCC, 1999). The concept of competence is fundamental to the autonomy and accountability of each healthcare professional and therefore to codes of conduct for health professionals (e.g. NMC, 2004a).

Current pre-registration nurse education curricula thus contain competencies under four 'domains', namely professional and ethical practices, care delivery, care management, and personal and professional development. 'Standards of proficiency' and outcomes are identified for 'entry to branch programmes' (i.e. outcomes for the CFP), and outcomes in each of the four domains for each of the four branches (mental health, adult, child and learning disabilities) for entry to the register, as noted in Chapter 2.

As we will see later it is absolutely vital for the mentor to establish very early during the clinical placement exactly which specific competencies they are expected to assess students on during that particular placement. Otherwise the assessment may not meet the curriculum requirements. In the notes you made in response to Activity 6.2, you may have mentioned that the NMC has already laid down the components that we need to assess in the form of competencies, but more detailed information can usually be found in a range of documents such as the student's course assessment booklet, the assessor's handbook, and the course curriculum.

You can obtain free hard copies of 'Standards of Proficiency' documents from the NMC or HPC, or print them from their Internet website, either to gain an overview, or for more detailed scrutiny of the standards and outcomes that pre-registration students have to achieve to be able to register in the relevant part of the Professional Register.

The NMC's (2004b) standards of proficiency and outcomes are further broken down into specific 'practice objectives' in the course curriculum. The outcomes and objectives for each module are discussed with students and mentors before the student embarks on the particular placement where they are expected to achieve them.

All assessments of the pre-registration curriculum are mandatory, and those in the CFP are set at academic level HE1 (or level C – certificate level); those for Year 2 are set at HE2 (level I – Intermediate or diploma level), and those for Year 3 at HE2 and

HE3 (level H – Honours degree level) depending on whether the student is following a diploma or a degree programme. Level M (Masters level), and level D (Doctoral level) are also identified. Various other ways of differentiating between academic levels have been developed recently, and in particular there are differences in the ways they are classified in the four UK countries.

The competencies booklet given to students contain other useful information such as the process of assessment, the roles and responsibilities of the mentor, those of the student, and the university support available to them.

### Optional activity – Pre-registration student assessment

Find out from your partner university all the assessments that the pre-registration student needs to pass for the branch programme appropriate to your clinical setting. You could access this information via the link tutor, for instance, for your clinical setting.

In addition to the placement competencies or practice objectives set by the university, students are encouraged to achieve as many other competencies as the placement can offer and thereby maximise learning. A number of clinical areas have their own clearly identified competencies or learning objectives that can be achieved during placement. A number of them are optional for pre-registration students but compulsory for newly appointed qualified healthcare professionals on induction or preceptee programmes.

  **Think Point 6.1 – Practice placement competencies**

Obtain a copy of the competencies or learning objectives for your practice area, and consider:

- Are these learning objectives separate from ward or team aims and objectives? If so, why?
- How far do the learning objectives give a clear indication of all competencies that students can learn during the placement?

The competencies are usually available in a 'learning resources' folder for students in your practice setting but it might prove useful to obtain a photocopy of this for yourself.

In addition to the regulatory bodies' standards of proficiency, professional bodies such as the Chartered Society for Physiotherapy publish further specific standards, such as those in the *Curriculum Framework for Qualifying Programmes in Physiotherapy*

(2002) for instance. This document identifies the nine outcomes that physiotherapy students have to achieve by the time they complete their preparatory programme, along with further guidelines. It specifies that, on successful completion of a recognised programme, graduates should be able to demonstrate their capacity to:

- practise within the core areas of physiotherapy;
- manage themselves and work with others to optimise results;
- enable people to optimise their health and social well-being;
- deliver physiotherapy in response to individual need;
- promote equality to all in physiotherapy practice;
- demonstrate and apply knowledge and understanding to issues affecting physio-therapy practice;
- engage in research and evidence-based healthcare;
- respond appropriately to changing demands;
- practise and promote CPD.

## Why Do We Need to Assess Our Students?

We have already referred to some of the aims of assessments. Most individuals have mixed feelings about being assessed, as on the one hand it creates anxiety, but on the other hand, on passing the assessment, the assessee can be given permission to practise the particular clinical skill without close supervision. To begin our discussion on why we need to assess, consider what the range of purposes of assessments is, in addition to the (NMC, 2006a) requirement for mentors to assess learners.

### Activity 6.3 – Purposes of assessments

Think of all the methods of assessment you noted in Activity 6.1, and of the reasons for assessing students and other learners. Make notes on these reasons. What did each assessment test?

As noted at the beginning of the chapter, according to the NMC the mentor must indicate that the student has achieved the NMC (2004b) standards of proficiency and is fit to practise, and thus the practice competencies are designed to test the student's ability to perform clinical patient care skills. Structured essays test the student's knowledge and understanding of concepts in nursing. In addition to these, assessments also ascertain learning in the affective domain (Bloom, 1956 – discussed in Chapter 3), that is, values and attitudes. Several purposes of assessments are identified by different writers. In summary, we assess learners:

- To establish and then authorise them as developing health professionals, to practise specific clinical skills without close supervision.
- To inform the learner of their level of achievement at that point in time.

- To determine the student's progress with the learning programme.
- To ascertain the learner's overall competence and fitness for practice.
- To motivate the learner towards new components of learning.
- To judge the level of professional learning in the cognitive (knowledge and thinking), psychomotor (dexterity with clinical skills), and affective (attitude) components.
- For the student to identify further learning needs based on self-assessment and mentor feedback.

As assessments also constitute an opportunity for identifying learning needs, this suggests that teaching and learning are integral components of the assessment process, and not simply a means of measuring attainment. Students are encouraged to undertake self-assessment and to reflect on their learning. It could be argued that all assessments are learning situations, in that if the assessee makes any error, then they are likely to be aware of it, or the assessor will point it out to them and identify learning needs. This notion also suggests that even if the student performs the skill competently, there is still scope for progressing from 'competent' to 'proficient' levels, for instance, and subsequently to 'expert' on Benner's (2001) skill acquisition continuum.

From the teacher's perspective, assessments also provide a measure of teaching effectiveness. It provides some feedback on the mentor's and their colleagues' effectiveness at teaching particular competencies during practice placements. Naturally, the student will normally have had some teaching related to those competencies at the university beforehand. Assessments of theory also provide nurse lecturers some measure of their university-based teaching.

In addition to the aims of assessments already mentioned, another function of assessments is to fulfil one of society's needs directly, in that they identify which healthcare professionals have acquired the necessary repertoire of knowledge and competencies for safe and competent practice, as a primary practitioner initially, and probably as a specialist later.

## Who Assesses Learners?

As to who assesses learners, obviously it is qualified healthcare professionals who have completed a mentoring course who are given 'a licence' to assess learners' competencies. However, it is pertinent to consider the broader question of who else are the relevant personnel to assess competencies.

 **Think Point 6.2 – Who assesses?**

Think about assessments you and your colleagues have been involved in recently. Spend a few minutes thinking about who conducted the assessments, on what, on whom and how. Is it only the mentor who assesses the learner's competencies, or are other individuals also involved?

Perhaps an immediate response to this Think Point is that it is the mentor who assesses, or teams of mentors. However, the NMC (2006a) indicates that assessments are also performed by other registrants, practice teachers and qualified teachers. In fact you might have concluded that all qualified healthcare professionals, including doctors, are involved in assessments, albeit often informally. So, the answer to the question 'Who assesses?' could be everyone in the clinical setting, but includes students' self-assessment, peer assessment, and assessment by patients or service users. These are now discussed.

## Student self-assessment

Self-assessment is one of the most valuable forms of assessment for students. It is almost always formative and therefore a learning exercise. As implied, the student uses a set of criteria or a checklist, written or mental, to self-assess their knowledge of a sub-topic area or of a specific competency. It also enables them to own the learning and to control the way they meet their needs. Self-assessment may be performed informally, or more formally by the use of profiling documents or reflective diaries.

Much informal or subconscious self-assessment carried out by learners is based on their own individual aspirations, values and beliefs. These could be influenced by their views on patient or service-user care based on their own personal and professional experiences.

## Activity 6.4 – Self-assessment

Take a critical look at the idea of self-assessment by students, and of the strengths and weaknesses of self-assessments, and identify as many of these as you can think of.

What is self-assessment? Falchikov (1986) states that in self-assessment the learner judges their own performance against their own assessment criteria. According to Boud (1991), self-assessment is characterised by involvement of students in identifying standards and/or criteria to apply to their work and making judgements about the extent to which they have met them.

On examining the concept with groups of post-registration students, a number of areas of strengths as well as weaknesses were identified (Gopee, 2000) – see Table 6.1.

## Peer assessment

The value and impact of peers' and colleagues' impressions of our competence in various aspects of our roles cannot be underestimated. This is often informal, with colleagues, friends and even family members having different perceptions of our capability, based perhaps on their different professional experiences.

**Table 6.1   The strengths and weaknesses of self-assessment**

| Strengths | Weaknesses |
|---|---|
| • Inspires a conscious effort to be honest with self<br>• Opportunity to identify limitations of own knowledge, and of learning needs<br>• Identify where more practice/knowledge is required<br>• Is less traumatic than traditional methods of assessment such as examinations | • Student can be too strict or too lenient<br>• Self-assessment is subjective and student may be unaware of the perceptions of relevant others<br>• Students may be unable to gauge the effectiveness of own performance<br>• Students can be too self-critical<br>• May worsen a student's poor self-image |

*Source*: Gopee (2000).

Because of its value to the student, increasingly peer assessment is being built into formal assessment processes. In distance and e-learning modes of education delivery, facilitators often encourage students to form own 'learning sets' for the purposes of learning together, discussions and questioning each other. Peer assessment, in this case, is not formal in that other students or colleagues do not usually award a summative 'pass' or 'fail' to the peer assessed. They do however provide valuable opinions and feedback on the individual's knowledge, which can be formally incorporated into a profile or a record of reflective learning. In this way peer assessment usually presents an opportunity to verbalise uncertainties and reservations about one's learning without having to deal with the anxiety of examinations and pass or fail situations.

Assessment by peers, formal or informal, is increasingly becoming accepted as an educationally sound activity. Many of us may find assessing our peers uncomfortable. We either do not wish to appear to be over-critical, and therefore tend not to assess or voice our views fully, or we feel that as we have such good rapport with our peers, we could damage their self-confidence with our 'criticisms'. It is also important to recognise that being assessed by our peer group can be more daunting than being assessed by a so-called expert. If it is done badly, peer assessment can quickly destroy students' confidence or make them feel unable to face their peers again.

Peer assessment, therefore, just like any other form of assessment, can benefit from the expertise of a facilitator if it is to be effective and help the student. Thus peers who are doing the assessing, as well the person being assessed, are helped by the facilitator to recognise the parameters of their roles. However, as with self-assessment, there can well be problematic areas related to peer assessment – Table 6.2 identifies some of the advantages and disadvantages.

Another related term is *peer review*, which involves seeking the views and impressions of peers in a structured or semi-structured way. When clinicians design a new protocol or audit tool for instance, they may ask an uninvolved colleague who works some distance away but in the same clinical specialism to comment on it prior to finalisation for use. Lecturers usually have to ask a colleague to observe their teaching on specified occasions and provide feedback against particular criteria. These are examples of peer review.

**Table 6.2    Advantages and disadvantages of peer assessment**

| Advantages | Disadvantages |
| --- | --- |
| • Confirms previously held belief in skills or lack of them<br>• Provides clarity to self-assessment findings<br>• Chance to share colleagues' experiences<br>• Identifying problems<br>• Receiving feedback<br>• Feedback from colleagues/students of equal status has impact<br>• Opportunity to practise the skill<br>• Is formative (i.e. is not a pass/fail mark for the course) | • Some can find it hard to take any criticism from equals<br>• Increased anxiety<br>• Someone can be over-critical and destructive<br>• Can be judgemental about the person<br>• Takes so much effort and resulting anxiety that pointed-out weaknesses may not be fully taken on board<br>• May not be supportive enough<br>• The individual might not accept peers' views<br>• Facilitators' knowledge of relevant literature, research, etc., may be limited<br>• Can destroy self-confidence and lead to deserting the venture/vocation altogether<br>• Disagreement between peers<br>• Availability of opportunities/peers for peer assessment<br>• Lack of commitment |

*Source*: Gopee (2001).

## Patient or service user involvement in assessment of competencies

One of the judges of how competently a healthcare professional learner performs a clinical skill could be the patient or service user. User involvement is increasingly advocated by regulatory bodies (e.g. NMC, 2006d). These entail patients or service users being involved in learner assessment and providing feedback on how competently the learner functioned in particular care interventions. Usually, the mentor gauges how content the patient or service user is with the care they receive by observation, and even by casually asking them. The patient or service user can provide feedback to the mentor about the assessee's communication skills, injection-giving skills, and teaching relaxation skills, for example.

In recommending user involvement in assessments, the NMC (2006d) advises HEIs to explore ways in which lay people (including service users and carers) can be involved in the assessment of practice, and supply evidence of this involvement, and of that of clinical practitioners in Programme Boards/Boards of Study that establish the requirements for practice learning and assessment.

## How are Assessments Conducted?

Learners deemed competent in performing a particular clinical skill can move on to learn other skills identified in their practice objectives for the placement. In this major section on how to assess, further principles of assessment are addressed, and comprise:

- ensuring the mentee has learned the clinical skill;
- key characteristics of assessors and essential interpersonal skills;
- dimensions of assessment;
- levels of assessment;
- fairness of assessment;
- assessment policies, approved strategies and performance criteria;
- validity and reliability of assessments.

Additionally, the process of assessment of competencies has to be managed, decisions made and feedback given to the assessee. These latter points, along with how the mentor averts and resolves problems of assessment, are examined in Chapter 7.

## Ensuring the mentee has learned the clinical skill

An important prerequisite of assessment of a learner is to ensure that they have been taught the clinical skill systematically and given the necessary practice opportunities over time and under supervision prior to the point of assessment. What skills, competence and competencies are was discussed in Chapter 2, and how learners acquire the required competencies, including stages and levels of skill acquisition (e.g. Benner, 2001; Fitts and Posner, 1973; Steinaker and Bell, 1979), in Chapter 3. But crucially and logically, before the student is asked to demonstrate that they are competent in any skill, they naturally need to learn to perform the skill according to approved procedures, and under the guidance of a registrant. The learning also has to be in the context of eventualities in the clinical setting.

## Key characteristics of assessors and essential interpersonal skills

Assessment is a role that has to be executed responsibly by the mentor. However, there are certain personal qualities and specific interpersonal skills that can ease the process for the learner. The former ENB (1994) identified specific or key characteristics of assessors and indicated that assessors should be able to demonstrate:

- A sound knowledge of, and skills in, contemporary nursing practice.
- A full understanding of the appropriate aspects of the curriculum.
- A commitment to create and maintain a supportive learning environment.
- The ability to apply the principles of teaching, supervising, facilitating and assessing in the practice setting.
- The ability to assess the level of attainment of criterion-based learning outcomes.
- Effective interpersonal skills within the tripartite relationship with students and patients or service users.
- The ability to facilitate alternative ways for the student to gain relevant experience and achieve the necessary learning outcomes.
- Effective collaboration with teacher colleagues.

## Activity 6.5 – Interpersonal skills in assessing a student

Make a list of what you consider to be the general communication skills required in all assessment situations, and then a list of the more specific communication skills required by the mentor for conducting assessments effectively.

Several communication skill items emerge when exploring in detail what and how the mentor communicates with the assessee. Box 6.1 lists many of the essential inter-personal skills that are required during assessments, identified by just one group of registrants on a mentor course.

---

### Box 6.1   Communication and interpersonal factors related to assessments

*Generic communication skills*

- Non-verbal communication – eye-contact, facial expression
- Body language – posture, body orientation, proximity, attitude, behaviour, space
- Being non-judgemental – warmth, empathy, respect
- Always remaining calm
- Openness
- Questioning – open or closed questions
- Reflecting
- Active listening
- Verbal communication – pace, volume, tone, clarity
- Diplomacy
- Considering environmental factors
- Being enthusiastic, interested
- Making time, using silence
- Constructive criticism/advice
- Approachable and friendly, non-intimidatory

*Specific interpersonal skills*

- Putting the assessee at ease
- If anxious, try and relax the assessee so they can show their true potential; build confidence by positive feedback if necessary
- Giving clear directions
- Continuous feedback
- Be non-judgemental by not criticising verbally or non-verbally
- If student's mind goes blank give clues/prompts
- Allowing enough time for the learner to perform the skill fully
- Making time to listen, and to maintain rapport
- Preventing observer bias and observer effect
- Ascertaining level of understanding of terminologies/jargon
- Confidence – in the student/in self
- Reinforcing what has been discussed

---

## Dimensions of assessment

There are a number of other essential facets of assessments that we need to consider to gain a more comprehensive picture of how to assess. Quinn and Hughes (2007) and others identify what is generally known as dimensions of assessments. Particularly relevant are whether assessments are:

- continuous or episodic;
- formative or summative;
- criterion-referenced or norm-referenced.

### Continuous or episodic assessments

Until the latter half of the 1980s, the assessment of pre-registration students used to take place at pre-determined points in their course. The student on the general nursing course was assessed on their ability to administer medications in Year 1 of the course, and to use aseptic techniques, and organise the total care of an individual or a group of patients or service users on specific subsequent occasions. They also had to pass written examinations at the end of the course. These are episodic assessments. Obviously students had to learn numerous other nursing skills necessary to function as a healthcare professional, which were identified in a booklet and signed as appropriate. Thus snapshot assessments were not seen as representing the wide range of skills acquired during placements, nor were they seen as a genuine representation of how students usually delivered care, and they therefore fell into disfavour. They were replaced by continuous assessment and subsequently by modularisation of preparatory programmes, involving assessment of practice and theory on numerous occasions throughout the course.

Episodic (or intermittent) assessments therefore involve testing the student at specific times or occasions during an educational programme, such as at the end of a module, a placement or year. Continuous assessment aims to increase the quality and quantity of evidence gathered in relation to achievement of competencies by each individual student. It involves a continuing awareness by the mentor of the student's level of knowledge and competence, and is thus a cumulative judgement about progress and achievement.

---

### Activity 6.6 – Advantages and disadvantages of continuous and episodic assessments

Consider what you think might be the advantages and disadvantages of episodic or continuous assessments, and make some notes.

---

The principal reason for episodic assessments being discredited in nursing and midwifery in the past is that decisions about the student's competence were being made on the basis of one-off performances. This performance, be it excellent or otherwise, might be atypical. Another disadvantage is that some key skills can remain untested if they do not present themselves during the identified assessment episode. Recently, following extensive consultation, the NMC (2006e) has introduced a point in the pre-registration nursing curriculum when 'essential skills clusters' need to be assessed by a 'sign-off mentor'. This is an example of episodic assessment and will be a requirement for registration with the NMC for students starting in September 2008.

*Formative or summative assessments*

Another dimension of assessment is whether an assessment is formative or summative. In common with the context of evaluation (which we discuss in Chapter 8), 'formative' relates to the development and improvement stages of something (e.g. a clinical skill). Its primary aim is to make the final performance as effective as possible. The basic goal of formative assessment is to promote learning and develop the student's ability under conditions in which they can experiment and think creatively in response to the course material, without being too concerned about grades. This applies to formative assessment of theory and of practical skills. In the latter the student has the opportunity to take time to learn the skill thoroughly with the support of mentors. Formative assessments are instituted to provide feedback to the student on their progress, and their aims therefore are to:

- maximise learning;
- identify strengths/weaknesses;
- inform the student of how they are progressing;
- allow for individual development.

'Summative' relates to a point in time during a unit of learning, for example a practice placement, when the mentor makes a decision about whether to declare the learner competent or otherwise on a specific component of the course. The ENB (1995: 5,10) indicated that a summative assessment is 'the judgement of student achievement of learning outcomes at appropriate stages of each programme, contributing to a grade and/or award'. They are conducted to determine whether the learner is now competent to work without direct supervision and, if so, then this is also recorded in their competencies' booklet.

Summative assessments also constitute a periodic record of the student's achievement of the aims and outcomes of a course or module. The grade awarded for these assessments, along with those for coursework and examinations contribute to the final classification of the student's university award.

It might prove useful to ask your mentee, or to look back on any long course you have done in recent years, and identify the range of formative and summative assignments incorporated in the programme. As to assessment in the clinical setting, the student learning part-skills (e.g. some of the skills of administering an intramuscular injection) actually constitutes a formative assessment. The NMC's (2006d) 'signing-off' of competencies point constitutes a summative assessment.

In healthcare courses, summative assessments are concerned with patient or service user safety and standards of practice. They are also concerned with justice for the student, and credibility of the university's awards. They must therefore meet the highest standards of reliability and validity, which are discussed in some detail later in this chapter.

*Criterion-referenced or norm-referenced assessments*

The third dimension of assessment we consider is norm referencing and criterion referencing. In norm-referenced assessment, the student's score, marks or grades are determined to an extent by those of other students in a given group or cohort. Programme Assessment Boards (also known as Award Boards) have the discretion to adjust the marks required by a particular cohort to achieve a particular grade if unusual circumstances have prevailed. Criterion-referenced assessments are different in that the score or mark given to a particular student for a particular piece of coursework is decided entirely on the basis of a pre-determined set of marking criteria. Students will have been informed of these criteria long before the assessment date.

---

:💡: **Think Point 6.3 – Norm- or criterion-referenced assessments**

Think about some of the assessments you've mentioned for Activity 6.1 and decide whether they are norm-referenced assessments or criterion-referenced.

---

Occasionally, a criterion-referenced assessment can be marked on a norm-referenced basis at the discretion of the appropriate Programme Assessment Board.

## Assessing different levels of competence

Student nurses tend to be taught and assessed at different academic levels during Year 1, Year 2 and Year 3. The NMC's standards of proficiency for CFP and branch programmes noted in Chapter 3 are configured at different academic levels in the competencies booklets that students take to practice placements. Healthcare assistants studying for national vocational qualification are also assessed differently at different levels.

To teach and assess competencies at different levels of learning, a number of current nurse education curricula tend to use Steinaker and Bell's (1979) model (or taxonomy) of experiential learning. This taxonomy consists of exposure level, participation, identification, internalisation and dissemination. A broad guide to how experiential taxonomy levels might equate with academic levels is:

- Certificate level/academic level 1 – exposure;
- Diploma level/academic level 2 – participation, identification and internalisation;
- Degree level/academic level 3 – dissemination.

This is a very simple classification and just a general guide which underpins specific wording of competencies to reflect the different levels. Alternatively, some programmes use Benner's (2001) stages of skill acquisition model, which was discussed in Chapter 2. Others use Bondy's (1983) five levels of competency, namely dependent, marginal, assisted, supervised and independent.

The assessment of theory of nursing on the other hand at different levels is usually based on Bloom's (1956) taxonomy of cognitive learning which was also discussed in Chapter 3. You may wish to look back to the appropriate section to remind yourself of the details of this model, which comprises knowledge, comprehension, application, analysis, synthesis, and evaluation. In both models of assessment, the first points, that is, exposure and knowledge, represent lower-level learning and the last points the higher levels.

## Fairness of assessments

In assessment we are measuring the performance of the individual student on particular competencies. Wouldn't you agree, however, that assessments have to be as objective as possible and must be fair to students? What does fairness of assessment mean?

## Activity 6.7 – Barriers to 'fairness'

Think about your own experiences of assessment (either assessing or being assessed) and consider instances that can make assessments 'unfair', and how we can make them 'fair'. Identify all factors that you feel interfere with the fairness of the assessment, using the three headings: (a) student factors; (b) mentor factors; and (c) environmental factors. If you can't remember being assessed, then make some notes of your own ideas of what we should be aware of during an assessment to ensure it is being conducted fairly.

It is conceivable that, on occasion, the demand being made on a student during assessment or the questions being asked may seem beyond the boundaries of what would generally be expected. Fairness of assessment refers to being aware of external circumstances that could influence the student's performance of the clinical skill. There are several factors that could hamper fairness of assessments. An unfair assessment could also mean that it might not be a valid assessment. Student factors that can make an assessment unfair include:

- expected level of knowledge is too high;
- theory–practice disjunction;
- not enough opportunities to practise the competencies;
- last-minute delays or changes;
- undeclared physical illness or fatigue.

You should be able to think of other student factors, including personal circumstances. Mentor factors include the mentor not working on the same shift as their mentee, bias towards or against the student, not having had educational preparation to become a mentor, overpowering attitude, and lack of knowledge of the student's course. Some of the factors in the clinical environment that might unfairly affect assessments are interruptions, lack of resources in clinical setting (e.g. equipment), suitability of placement and low staffing levels.

## Pass or fail: performance criteria

Following a fairly conducted assessment, the mentor has to decide whether it's a pass or a fail for the particular competencies. This decision may well depend entirely on whether the student followed the trust's approved procedure closely to perform the clinical skill, or the written (or unwritten) protocol. The procedure is the main form of 'performance criterion'.

---

**Think Point 6.4 – What am I looking for in the student?**

Consider two examples of assessment of competence that you may have been involved in. This could be a pre-registration or post-registration course competency.

(a)   How did the mentor determine what criteria to use to pass or fail the learner?
(b)   What influenced them to choose these particular criteria?

---

The term *performance criteria* refers to the pre-determined set of components that are used for deciding whether the learner performed the clinical skill competently. They can therefore constitute a checklist of the step-by-step actions taken by the assessee when performing the skill. These step-by-step actions are normally the trust's approved procedure for that skill, and are set down in two columns as 'actions' and 'rationales', and usually supported by references to make them evidence based. They are normally kept in the clinical setting's 'Policies and Procedures' section for use and for reference purposes. There is likely to be a separate folder for clinical guidelines or protocols which refer to expanded role competencies.

The term performance criteria is also used in NVQ programmes but with a slightly different meaning. Quinn and Hughes (2007) refer to them as *performance indicators*. However, for those nursing activities for which there is no identified step-by-step approved procedure, the performance criteria can be established by asking the skilled practitioner to describe to someone in detail everything that they would do to perform the skill competently. For instance, there might not be a procedure for assessing communication skills, for bed-making, for taking body temperature using tympanic thermometers or, say, for doing patient handovers. A set of performance criteria for patient handovers (or 'reporting on patients' progress') is presented in Box 6.2.

---

**Box 6.2   Performance criteria for assessing competency – patient handover**

- Have the right documentation (e.g. care plan/pathway) to refer to
- Have a good understanding of the patient's conditions
- State the procedures that have been performed (e.g. removal of drains, sutures, etc.)
- Keep the information concise and focused
- Use appropriate language

*(Continued)*

- Pitch the amount of information imparted to the level of knowledge the handover recipients already have (e.g. more detailed information may need to be given if new staff or students are present)
- Ensure that all necessary information is given
- Inform of individual patient's overall progress
- Note any relevant communication from the patient's family, or from members of the multi-disciplinary team
- State any investigation results received, and any subsequent action prescribed
- State any changes in medication, and patient's reaction to them
- State the plan of care for the rest of the day
- Include patient's awareness of own condition (e.g. in mental health)
- Observe confidentiality issues, especially for bedside handovers

For competencies for which there are no written performance criteria in the clinical setting in the procedures or clinical guidelines folder, they might be found in, for instance, *The Royal Marsden Hospital Manual of Clinical Nursing Procedures* (Dougherty and Lister, 2006). They might also be available from the National Institute of Clinical Excellence (NICE), especially clinical guidelines, via their website or from manufacturers' instructions. As in the trust's procedure, clinical guidelines are usually tabulated as actions and rationales in two columns, and include a reference list. However, from the time a book or clinical guideline is written to the time it is available for use, adjustments may have been made to the procedure, based on more up-to-date evidence or research. Trust-based procedures tend to have an addendum to reflect this, which in fact makes them even more up to date than books.

As to keeping the information precise, Castledine (1998), for instance, indicates that handover reports are time limited as they could be seen as keeping healthcare staff away from direct patient care. On noticing ineffective patient handovers practices, Davies and Priestley (2006) suggest that conversation on irrelevant topics should be excluded from this exercise. Furthermore, some commentators like Walsh and Ford (1989) see handovers as a ritual, although in reality they are a necessary medium for communicating the effects of care and treatment to staff on the next shift.

Depending on the clinical specialism, further specific information may need to be imparted during handovers, for example resuscitation status, mobility levels in rehabilitation services. Very importantly, often teaching and learning points arise from patient handovers, for both students and clinically based unqualified staff and registrants. Thus the performance criteria for passing or failing a student on their ability to do patient's handover can be quite involved.

## Validity and Reliability of Assessments

The principles of assessment constitute further key considerations that are usually referred to as attributes or essential factors. There are four attributes that are absolutely crucial in all assessment of competencies. These are (a) validity, (b) reliability, (c) discrimination, and (d) practicability (or usability) of assessments.

## Validity

Validity is the most crucial aspect of an assessment in that it refers to the extent to which the assessment measures what it is expected to measure. A valid assessment is one that assesses the competency or learning outcome(s) it set out to assess, and not target other competencies that might not have been learnt adequately at that point in time. The five main types of validity are content validity, predictive validity, concurrent validity, construct validity and face validity, but some of these apply more to the overall curriculum, than just to assessment of competencies in the clinical setting.

### Content validity
This refers to the extent to which the assessment samples adequately the content of the curriculum. Do the assessment question and assignment guidelines assess all the learning outcomes of the curriculum? Note that for various reasons not everything the student learns during the course can be assessed. Content validity is primarily addressed by the structure of the assessment and is monitored by the programme manager for the course.

### Predictive validity
This is about to the extent to which the result can predict the future performance of the student. It is important for the mentor to determine if the student's performance during, say, a particular practical assessment, can predict how far he or she will perform to the same standard in future situations, and also whether they can adjust the performance to different clinical settings, for example, from a ward setting to community care, and to different patients.

### Concurrent validity
This refers to the extent to which the assessment results correlate with those of other assessments administered at the same time. In other words, if two different assessments are designed to measure the same learning outcomes, then the student should do equally well in both, for example asking a student to talk through how they would perform a skill, and to actually demonstrate it.

### Construct validity
Validity that refers to the extent to which the results of the assessment are related to impressions or evidence gained from observations of the individual's behaviour with regard to their attitudes, values and intelligence (which are also known as psychological constructs) is referred to as construct validity.

### Face validity
Face validity involves stopping to consider the overall impression about how competently the clinical skill was performed, and whether the student actually demonstrates the complex array of observational, analytical, interpersonal and technical skills required for the competency.

**Think Point 6.5 – Types of validity**

A first-year student is being assessed on a surgical ward changing a patient's dressing using aseptic technique. The purpose of this particular episode of assessment is specifically with regards to changing a dressing using aseptic technique skills. However, during the procedure the patient makes some statements that clearly reflect marked disorientation, and the student is unable to respond therapeutically to disorientation. The aseptic technique is performed correctly. Should the mentor pass or fail the student? Which decision is the valid decision?

## Reliability

In addition to validity, another key consideration of any assessment is its reliability, which is a term that is used to indicate the consistency with which an assessment measures what it is designed to measure. This means that if the assessment is conducted again, the same level of performance should produce the same result, provided other variables remain similar.

To take this a step further, reliability has to do with consistency in the grade or result awarded for a particular piece of work:

(a) between different mentors;
(b) between different occasions on which the work is done; and
(c) between different methods of assessment

In all cases, the result or grades awarded should be almost or preferably exactly the same for the test to be deemed 'reliable'. The NMC (2006d) indicates that programme providers should supply evidence of monitoring:

- effective inter/intra-mentor reliability of practice assessment;
- robust moderation of practice assessment;
- external examiners report fully on practice learning and assessment.

**Think Point 6.6 – Reliability of assessments**

Think about assessments you or your colleagues have been involved in recently. Then spend a few minutes thinking about how reliably the assessment was conducted. Decide why you think the assessment was or was not reliable.

Generally, there are certain factors that might negatively affect reliability being achieved. These are practical issues such as:

- individual biases;
- halo effect;
- insufficient time allocated for the assessment;
- ambiguity of questions being asked;
- competence as an assessor;
- whether more than one assessor was involved, as two assessors could mean less subjectivity;
- whether the performance criteria had been agreed.

## Discrimination

Discrimination in assessment refers to the ability of assessment to differentiate between different levels of competence demonstrated by students, such as Year-1 students, Year 2 or 3. Steinaker and Bell's (1979) taxonomy of learning is generally used to differentiate between these levels of competences. However, by and large, learners should be given the opportunity to demonstrate their true level of ability, regardless of the level he/she is expected to reach at the particular stage of the course.

Discrimination also refers to the distinction between all learners. A healthcare assistant would be assessed against different criteria for a particular clinical skill, from a medical student, or from a student nurse, for instance, mainly because the level of theoretical knowledge expected of each is different.

## Practicability (or usability)

This concept refers to whether the assessment can be conducted within the time and with the resources available.

---

 **Think Point 6.7 – Practicability of assessments**

Think about your own practice setting. Have you encountered situations when you are required to assess a learner's competencies but felt that the time allocated was not adequate or that it was not practical to conduct the assessment comprehensively?

---

Mentors encounter problems of practicability of assessment when practice placements are too short, or when for some reason the assessments have been left until the last few days of the placement. In the study of assessment of competence by Phillips et al. (2000) several problems of practicability of assessment were identified. The more crucial ones will be explored in Chapter 7.

## Implementing Approved Assessment Procedures

Each university identifies clearly in their course documents exactly which assessments students have to pass to complete the course successfully. This is supported by further assessment guidelines and specifications on how students are to acquire the necessary knowledge and competence to do so. Examples of course assessments were cited at the beginning of this chapter in response to Activity 6.1.

The procedure for assessing practice competencies is detailed in students' placement booklets. These procedures, alongside other requirements for the course will have been planned before the course starts, under the scrutiny of the university's quality assurance guidelines and protocols for designing courses and modules. Thereafter, they will have gone through a rigorous course approval process before being offered to students.

The pass marks for assessments may vary by a few marks between different universities, as may the weightings between practical and theoretical assessments, or different assessment components. The number of assessments may vary, as may the number of formative assessments related to the summative ones. Each course and module is assessed on its learning outcomes, indicative content and competencies.

All universities are governed by identified boards and committees for addressing specifically designated functions related to the courses they offer. An example of a university-level board is the Academic Board and that of a committee is the Deferral Committee. Those at faculty, school or department level include the Board of Study and the Subject Assessment Board.

The functions of each of these committees, whose membership includes clinical managers, the subject librarian, the placement manager, for instance, and boards, are identified in their terms of reference. The Faculty's Board of Study for pre-registration courses, for instance, holds meetings each term to receive module and programme results, module and practice placement evaluations, and issues raised at course consultative committee meetings. The mentor is not required to know in detail what each committee does, unless they are members of those committees, but some of the decisions made by these committees may affect mentoring activities with students during practice placement, such as extending the placement.

The university's Board of Study fulfils essential functions, in that it assumes ultimate responsibility for the effective delivery, evaluation and revision of modules, courses and the students' programmes of studies, some of the feedback for which it receives from relevant Faculty Board(s). It tends to have an overall monitoring role in relation to module or course assessments. During the planning stages, the modules will have been fully discussed by the Course or Module Curriculum Planning Teams. They will have been designed following the university's protocol. It would for instance have followed the university's protocol for writing modules, and the university's Assessment Parity Rules, which include rules on word limits for courseworks. They would then have been approved by an assembled panel of experts, which usually includes representations from the NMC, probably the HPC, and subject specialists from other universities. In addition to the overall university assessment strategy there are specific assessment strategies within each course and module, thereby ensuring that each programme is fully structured before students start on the course.

## Policies and strategies for assessments

Students' practice placement competencies booklets clearly identify the procedure for assessment of competencies. This entails an initial mentor–mentee interview when the competencies to be achieved are ascertained, and often a learning contract constituted. Approximately halfway through the placement a mid-placement interview takes place to ascertain the student's progress with the contracted competencies. During the last week of the placement a final interview is conducted to ascertain which clinical competencies have been achieved, and those that have are signed and dated accordingly.

All aforementioned proceedings are documented as evidence of progress with continuous assessment, for the final summative assessment of the practice module and for legal reasons. The practice competencies' booklets also identify the exact roles and responsibilities of the mentor, those of the student before, during and after the placement. They also contain a set of components related to the student's professionalism, attitude and their teamworking, and which the student must demonstrate at a satisfactory level (related to construct validity). Usually there is also a section on actions to take regarding under-achieving students.

## Chapter Summary

This chapter has focused on assessment of learners' clinical knowledge and competence, answering questions about what assessments are, why we conduct them, who assesses, and when and how? Having completed this chapter you will have learnt about:

- What the term assessment means, in the context of assessing professional knowledge and competence. This involved considering various definitions of assessments, and the exact competencies to be assessed.
- Why we need to assess our students and learners, that is, the exact purposes and aims of assessments, and at which particular points in students' programmes of study to assess.
- Who assesses learners, including student self-assessment, and peer assessment, and patient or service user involvement in assessment of competencies.
- How assessments are conducted, which includes ensuring the mentee has learned the clinical skill; the key characteristics of assessors including essential interpersonal skills; and the dimensions of assessments, which includes continuous or episodic assessments, formative or summative and criterion- or norm-referenced. Assessing different levels of competence, fairness of assessments and the use of performance criteria.
- Validity, reliability, discrimination and practicability as essential aspects of assessments, and the role of approved assessment policies, procedures and strategies.

# SEVEN

# Leadership and the Challenges of Mentoring

## Introduction

Mentors are generally informed of the learner allocated to them well before the placement starts, to which the mentor responds by structuring a plan of learning experiences for the learner for the duration of the placement. This chapter focuses on the mentor's leadership in forward planning, and in encountering the challenges of mentoring, and therefore covers:

- The mentor's leadership in forward planning for mentoring and assessing competence.
- Averting or resolving potential and actual problems of assessment of competence, action plans for learning, and reassessment.
- Responsibilities and accountability of the mentor, including ethical and legal aspects of mentoring, and how mentors can ascertain intra- and inter-mentor reliability of the assessments they conduct.
- Supporting the struggling or under-achieving student through planned actions for effective learning, and helping them as appropriate.

Research findings (e.g. Phillips et al., 2000; Duffy, 2004) highlight various day-to-day problems that could be encountered by both mentors and students in the assessment of students' competencies during practice placements. Assessments are conducted 'on the hoof' by registrants the assessee 'bumps into', and as part of several other roles were issues highlighted by Phillips et al. (2000); 'failure to fail' was the main problem highlighted by Duffy (2004). The NMC (2006a: 56), under the leadership domain, indicates that mentors should 'demonstrate leadership skills for education within practice and academic settings'. The outcomes for mentors associated with leadership competence are:

- Plan a series of learning experiences that will meet students' defined learning needs.
- Be an advocate for students to support them accessing learning opportunities that meet their individual needs, involving a range of other professionals, patients, clients and carers.
- Prioritise work to accommodate support of students within their practice roles.
- Provide feedback about the effectiveness of learning and assessment in practice.

These outcomes reflect the mentor's leadership in the context of planning for the placement, supporting, prioritising and giving feedback. As for planning 'learning experiences' and 'accessing learning opportunities', these components were discussed in Chapter 1 to some extent, but in Chapter 4 in particular. Careful forward planning of own work and prioritising are key features of the mentor's leadership role towards achievement of placement competencies, along with acting proactively to avert the likely contemporary problems of assessments, and dealing with those that do occur. At the end of the assessment, the mentor has to inform the student of their levels of achievement, and of their decision to award the student a pass or fail for that assessment component. It is in relation to assessment of competence that mentors encounter most of the challenges to their role.

## Chapter outcomes

On completion of this chapter you should be able to:

1. Explain how forward planning and prioritising work are important ways in which the mentor exercises leadership.
2. Identify likely problems of assessment of competencies, and how the mentor averts or resolves them.
3. Present an analysis of the responsibilities and accountability of the mentor in the assessment of practice competencies, along with related ethical and legal aspects of mentoring.
4. Ascertain the mentor's role in supporting the struggling student, and the use of various resources and guidelines in doing so.

Leadership as a notion in its own right was referred to in Chapter 5 in the context of healthcare professionals acting as agents in the management of change (see Table 5.2 for the approaches taken by transactional and transformational leaders). For a thorough and up-to-date analysis of leadership, the reader is referred to Kouzes and Posner's *The Leadership Challenge* (2003).

## The Mentor's Leadership in Managing Assessments

Assessment of competencies at times involves one-off short episodes of direct observation of the learner performing clinical skills using the trust's procedure. Otherwise, it is a continual process occurring throughout the practice placement. Assessment of theory is conducted and managed by the university through coursework essays and written examinations, and the process of assessment of students' competencies has to be managed by the mentor.

The various problems that are likely to be associated with assessments make early and careful planning of assessment imperative. Such planning constitutes an endeavour to ensure that the learner achieves the identified learning objectives for the placement, and to pre-empt problems. There is also the danger that if interruptions do occur during episodes of assessment, then the mentor could miss vital steps in the performance of the skill and decide on a pass (or fail) with insufficient information. Incorrect or unsafe practice can be missed.

## Managing the process of assessment in the clinical setting

### Activity 7.1 – Planning and managing the process of assessment of practice

This activity asks you to explore in detail how to manage the assessment of competencies or skills. To do this, focus on the specified outcomes or competencies of a specific section of the pre-registration course for your healthcare profession (e.g. NMC's, 2004b outcomes for entry to the branch programme) or the outcomes of a post-registration healthcare course. These will normally be found in the student's practice outcomes or competencies booklet.

   You might choose to work with a colleague or course peer who is in a similar specialism as you on this activity. Identify in detail everything that needs to be done to begin and complete the assessment of these competencies, from the time the student starts on the clinical placement to when the student is signed as competent for particular competencies. Include everything such as how you'd ensure the skills (or knowledge/attitude) have been learnt, and organisational aspects that have to be considered to ensure the assessment proceeds as planned.

From your response to Activity 7.1, you would have verbalised various preparations needed to ensure assessment of competencies is completed effectively. For all assessments there are usually certain curriculum regulations that need to be adhered to, such as assignment submission dates and the procedure to follow if the student is referred. A number of key points specifically related to managing practical assessments are identified in Box 7.1.

---

**Box 7.1   Planning and managing the assessment process**

In sequence

| | |
|---|---|
| Prior to the assessment | • Agree, during Week 1 of placement, the objectives/competencies that need to be achieved and assessed. |
| | • Ensure the learner has learnt the skill, allocate registrants to teach the skill in accordance with agreed performance criteria. The skill is taught at the appropriate academic level. The learner is given sufficient practice opportunities and has been formatively assessed during the placement. |

*(Continued)*

---

*(Continued)*

| | |
|---|---|
| | • Mentor feels (a) up to date with skills being assessed; (b) competent to assess/has attended mentor update course (c) takes a supportive and positive approach. |
| | • Day of assessment – ensure the student feels ready for the assessment, set time of day, consider 'practicability' and fairness of assessment issues. |
| | • Colleagues aware if and when they can interrupt (if necessary). |
| | • If on call, advise switchboard who to divert your calls to. |
| | • Agree performance criteria. |
| During the assessment | • Use appropriate communication skills (see Box 6.1). |
| | • Create a climate that enables the student to relax so that they can perform the skill to the best of their ability. |
| | • Safety issues – if assessee makes a mistake consider seriousness of mistake and intervene, or provide prompt/clues, as appropriate. |
| | • Responsive assessment (Neary, 2000b), taking into account the patient's changing healthcare needs. |
| | • Situated assessments, in the context of available resources, and clinical activities, for instance. |
| | • Consider predictive validity of assessments, that is, whether the assessee can perform as well in future and in other patient-care situations. |
| After the assessment | • Need to exercise professional judgement throughout. |
| | • Decide on whether to award a pass or fail for each skill or competency. |
| | • Give feedback according to established good practice (discussed next). |
| | • Ensure documentation is complete – for clinical intervention, student competency, and of feedback given. |
| | • If fail is awarded, then the mentor needs to follow the university's procedure, which normally includes informing the link tutor or practice educator. |

## Making decisions and giving feedback to the assessee

Following assessment of competency, the mentor has to indicate to the assessee whether they have passed or failed. Prior to this, however, the mentor needs to give feedback to the assessee on their performance of the clinical skill because all assessments should be learning situations, and the feedback should motivate the assessee to reflect on how to improve performance, or build on a good performance. Feedback is also a means of justifying the pass or fail result. Feedback can be: (a) *intrinsic feedback,* which occurs within the performer through self-assessment and reflection or (b) *extrinsic feedback* (or augmented feedback), given by the assessor or peers and done concurrently during the skill performance, and/or on completion of the performance. Some mentors find it difficult to give honest feedback on a weak or faulty student performance. This could be tricky for the assessee as well, but feedback has to be given honestly, and is generally accepted more readily if given constructively.

It is useful to ask the assessee how they felt they performed straight (or soon) after completion of the clinical skill, instead of telling them first how well or badly they performed. The benefits of asking the student are that this is likely to make them put aside any anxiety they might still have about their performance, think more objectively, and be more receptive to feedback. So, the mentor could ask, 'How do you think you did?' This constitutes self-assessment by the learner (which was discussed in Chapter 6), which should also give the mentor an indication of the learner's insights into their level of competence. Good practice guidelines for giving feedback to students are listed in Box 7.2.

---

### Box 7.2   Guidelines for giving feedback to the student after clinical skill performance

- Ensure privacy and that adequate time is allocated.
- Use the sandwich method, which entails starting with comments on the positive points or strengths, discussing areas for improvement, and ending on positive notes.
- Give feedback constructively, as the aim of feedback is to enable the learner to learn and improve.
- Be sensitive to the recipient's feelings and self-esteem throughout this exercise.
- Try to be honest and fair but never be destructive.
- Be clear and concise.
- Allow the recipient of the feedback time to discuss and ask for clarification.
- Do not allow anxiety levels to increase unduly.
- Treat the recipient as an individual, and focus upon behaviour rather than personality traits.
- Acknowledge good practice.
- Suggest measures to correct inappropriate practice.
- Remain calm and objective; do not respond in kind to anger, aggression and defensiveness.
- Motivate the recipient to consolidate strengths and address limitations through strategies such as action plans.
- Be empowering through encouragement of the recipient to comment and expand upon issues raised.

*Source:* adapted from Egan (2002).

Good general communication skills are essential when giving feedback, including non-verbal communication such as maintaining eye contact. The RCN (2005a) notes that following feedback, action plans or learning points should be mutually agreed. However, in an ethos of self-directed learning, ultimately it is up to the receiver of the feedback to decide how much to heed and act upon, and when, and to be accountable for their decisions.

## Good practice guidelines for assessments

This section builds on the important principles of assessment of clinical skills performance discussed in Chapter 6, and in some current literature such as ENB/DoH (2001b) and Rowntree (1987). A set of guidelines for the day-to-day mechanics of assessment is therefore constituted and presented in Box 7.3.

---

**Box 7.3    Good practice guidelines for the day-to-day mechanics of assessment**

- Allocate mentors for teaching specific skill/knowledge
- Utilise opportunities for formative assessments
- Arrange time and date, and diary it; treat it as 'protected time' (e.g. DoH, 1999; NMC, 2006d)
- Inform other staff to ensure they do not interrupt (considering staffing levels of course)
- Inform patient and obtain permission for student assessment
- Ensure all equipment is available
- Ensure assessee has had opportunity to practise the skill
- Ensure mentor is fully available
- Be sensitive to the student's self-confidence or lack of it
- Be aware of any crises in the clinical setting (e.g. staff sickness, stress)
- Plan the assessment, ensuring availability of procedures and guidelines
- Take safety measures if required

- Create opportunity for learner to talk through the procedure, if necessary
- Always remain calm
- If the assessee displays awe of the assessor – give confidence
- Beware of unachievable goals
- Look enthusiastic and motivated
- Allow student to work at own pace
- Allow for holistic care
- Ensure assessee knows the performance criteria for the skill
- Allow reflection and give feedback
- Use professional judgement
- Be aware of other factors (e.g. learner being preoccupied with assignments)
- Heed criticisms of assessments such as research findings such as 'failing to fail' (Duffy, 2004), and 'on-the-hoof' assessments (Phillips et al., 2000)

---

*(Continued)*

- Work in teams as this strengthens the reliability of assessments.
- Seek the opinions of colleagues who have experience of working with the learner being assessed, when feasible

- Intervene appropriately if unsafe practice is about to occur
- Do not be biased by occasional polarised instances of exceptionally thorough or poor practice
- Document results as required by the assessment strategy

Various viewpoints discussed so far suggest that appropriate documentation is vital to mentoring activities. In fact, documentation of assessments is crucial, considering the NMC's (2005a) indication that what is not recorded should be treated as not having been performed.

## Activity 7.2 – The student's practice competencies

Look through your copy (mentor's copy) or the student's copy of the practice competencies booklet, and read the sections where it identifies the roles of the mentor, the link tutor and personal tutor, and of the student during the placement.

A clause in the booklet also usually states the actions that the mentor needs to take if the mentee is perceived as underachieving or 'failing'. This tends to entail drawing on the expertise and functions of the link tutor, the practice educator or the student's personal tutor. There is also a section on the appeals procedure. However, for each new course or module being offered, there would have been a briefing session for prospective mentors so that they become familiar with the course requirements, the specific competencies to be achieved, and any other issues.

If you are on a mentoring course yourself, it is very important that, on completion of the course, before you conduct any student assessment, you acquaint yourself with the student's placement competencies, and preferably the overall assessment strategy for the course. Furthermore, you should fully understand the particular summative assessment that you are going to conduct. The action to take in case of 'failure to achieve required standard' by the learner, and the 'appeals procedure' are discussed later in this chapter. The importance of careful forward planning to ensure assessments of practice competencies proceed systematically during practice placement, prevents problems surfacing, maximises learning, and reduces the likelihood of the student experiencing undue stress, is extremely important.

Despite careful planning, unfolding day-to-day events could still disrupt the smooth running of assessments. The patient could refuse consent to students performing skills on them, staff sickness, unexpected emergency admissions or referrals might present as obstacles. However, these do not always present as problems, as Neary (2000a), Philips et al. (2000), and others recommend 'responsive assessment', which includes taking into account situational contexts such as prevailing resource issues, and the patient's current physiological or psychological state. Furthermore, as far as possible, mentors and their managers should endeavour to quantify and allocate 'protected time' for mentoring.

### Intra- and inter-mentor reliability

Mentor preparation courses usually also incorporate an exploration of how intra- and inter-mentor reliability are monitored after qualifying as a mentor, especially in relation to conducting assessments. This has been identified as an essential mentor activity previously by the ENB (1997) (referred to as intra- and inter-assessor reliability), and currently of course by the NMC (2006d).

The term *intra-mentor reliability*, in the mentor's assessment role, refers to how consistently the mentor assesses particular categories of students on particular clinical skills, that is, that he or she uses the same identified performance criteria for a skill, within a responsive assessment approach. *Inter-mentor reliability* refers to the consistency with which all mentors assess a particular category of students on particular clinical skills.

---

### Think Point 7.1 – Intra- and inter-mentor reliability

Think of ways in which mentors can achieve and monitor intra- and inter-mentor reliability. What are the informal and more structured situations or opportunities that they can utilise to explore these?

---

As you would have sensed, intra- and inter-mentor reliability refer to all roles of the mentor, such as those enunciated in the eight NMC (2006a) domains, associated competences and outcomes for the mentor, although it is usually related to assessments. There are various ways of monitoring intra- and inter-mentor reliability. One of the most effective of these is through discussion groups or workshops on annual mentor update study days. All mentors are required to attend these updates to remain on the university's or trusts' local register (or database) of current mentors (ENB, 1997; NMC, 2006d). The update study days and trust-based mentor update sessions provide a suitable opportunity to raise any issues and also to explore consistency within and across mentors. Case studies can be explored in small groups, or these groups can be invited to discuss them in the context of situations they've personally encountered as mentors. In these groups consistency in assessment by each mentor and between mentors can be explored, and, with the help of the facilitator, benchmarks of good practice can be established.

However, monitoring intra- and inter-mentor reliability mustn't wait for update study days. Informal monitoring is undertaken continuously through discussions with peers or team members in the clinical setting or unit, with one's line manager, or the mentor's own mentor or clinical supervisor.

Further ways of achieving intra-mentor reliability are by:

- Consistently using approved protocols/clinical guidelines.
- Ascertaining that approved procedures and clinical guidelines are up to date.
- Ensuring own competence and skills are up to date.
- Informal monitoring of own pass/fail rates of mentees.
- Ensuring appropriate environment for assessing, for example, the transferability of competence from skills laboratories to different care settings (i.e. community, critical care).
- Ensuring the learner is being taught to the same standard and protocol/procedure by different registrants/associate mentors.
- Student feedback such as evaluating how the student feels about the assessment process and decisions.
- External feedback, from colleagues through reflections on assessments conducted.
- Ensuring learners are aware of level of performance expected of them.
- Reflection-on-action on assessment just conducted.
- Ensuring being aware of halo effect, being non-judgemental, for instance about the assessee as a person; objectivity.
- Being consistent in own standard of clinical practice.

Other ways of achieving inter-mentor reliability are by:

- Mentor meetings within ward/unit team – formal and informal.
- Involving practice educator when uncertain.
- Consulting colleagues on same ward/unit as appropriate.
- Auditing mentor's performance of assessments (e.g. by negotiating peer assessment).
- Student feedback about mentor's practice setting.
- Feedback from university following student evaluations.
- Monitoring attendance at mentor updates, trust-based or university-based.
- Knowing and using link tutor.
- Exploring at clinical supervision meetings.
- Ensuring same clinical guidelines/protocols were being used.
- Monitoring mentors are up to date with clinical skills.

## Averting and Resolving Problems of Assessments

Potential problems of assessment of practice competencies can be averted by careful planning, and this is the component wherein the mentor's leadership is absolutely essential. However, problems with assessments do occur and, when they do, they have to be treated as a component of mentoring, and resolved, and endeavour to learn from them.

### Potential problems of assessment of competence

The aims or purposes of assessments are quite clearly identified by several writers on nurse education, as noted under 'Why do We Need to Assess our Students?' in Chapter 6. However, how far and how smoothly these aims are achieved in reality varies. We also need to consider exactly what the problems that mentors encounter in the assessment of students are, and what the criticisms directed at assessments are, including those of written examinations.

## Activity 7.3 – Current problems of assessments

- Think of the weaknesses of assessments and reasons why assessments, even written examinations, are unpopular with students (assuming they are). Make brief notes.
- Identify the actual problems that tend to occur with student assessment of theory and practice in your healthcare profession, ones that you have experienced or observed, or that you feel could occur.

Mentors and learners experience various difficulties with assessment of practice competencies. For assessment of theoretical knowledge (e.g. of human physiology) and numerical skills as in drug administration and nurse prescribing courses, written examinations remain a favoured method, particularly in higher education. The likely solutions to the problems that you have identified will be explored shortly. A range of problems of assessments was identified by just one group of students on a mentoring course. These are presented in Box 7.4.

---

### Box 7.4   Problems with assessments

- Leaving things to the last minute (i.e. poor time planning)
- Difficulty with integration of theory and practice, or ineffective application
- Personality problems/clashes
- Problems of organisation in the clinical setting
- Lack of time
- Student disagrees with mentor
- Attitude problems – student's or mentor's
- Structure of learning programme (e.g. placement is too short)

- Mentor accountable and responsible for how student performs clinical skills
- Inconsistency of student performance
- Student absence
- Mentor low morale
- Mentor changes or is absent
- Student appears indifferent
- Student's level of knowledge
- Lack of resources (e.g. equipment)
- Non-co-operation or refusal of consent by the patient or service user

---

One of the most cited difficulties mentors face is insufficient time for mentoring activities. Cognisance of this recurrent problem necessitates more robust leadership on the part of the mentor in terms of forward planning, prioritising and proactive actions. The empirical study on assessments by Phillips et al. (2000) highlighted various problems encountered by assessors, which are:

1. The quality of assessment varies enormously, depending on staffing levels and workload in the clinical setting.
2. Named assessors perform their assessor role as one of many other essential roles.
3. Many assessments are performed informally by registrants the assessee 'bumps into' during the course of their duty (i.e. 'opportunistic' and 'piecemeal').
4. Few assessment schedules recognise theories derived from day-to-day 'real' clinical practice, and remain a problem for assessors.
5. A major part of registrants' practice involves solving the operational and ethical dilemmas they regularly face in 'situations' with competing demands on their time.
6. The most valid assessments are those of (a) 'situated understanding' (explained under 8) and (b) judgement that occurs as a result of close observation of the assessee over a sustained period by the assessor.
7. Nursing and midwifery practice has to meet the expectations of a wide range of stakeholders, including individual patients and relatives, individual practitioners, user groups, Trusts, HEIs, Strategic Health Authorities, the healthcare professions regulatory bodies and the Department of Health.
8. The conditions under which assessees are assessed are variable but should always be 'situated' and therefore take into account the constraints and possibilities in the clinical setting.
9. Mentors experience difficulty in ascertaining different levels in practice, except for periodically considering current and alternative modes of practice.
10. Few assessors feel well prepared for doing assessments and most express a desire for continuing support after initial preparation, and consideration of adequate infrastructure for valid and reliable assessments.

An earlier study conducted by Satterly (1981) highlighted weaknesses with assessments that can still occur, and can arise across academic subjects. Satterly identified several 'objections to assessments', such as assessments being limited to relatively trivial educational objectives while the most important aims of education are inaccessible to testing. He suggested that some types of assessments constitute an invasion of privacy of the individual, that assessments encourage pupils to develop the styles of thought or intellectual 'tricks' required by tests and not the skills the education institution wishes them to achieve.

Many of these weaknesses could occur in healthcare courses, although actions have since been taken to remedy some of them. For instance, with regards to assessments being limited to relatively trivial educational objectives, and ignoring more important aims of education, a curriculum that is too focused on assessment of specific objectives could overlook some of the more important aims of education. Entwistle (1994) identifies the aims of higher education as:

- Adopting a distinctive way of thinking about concepts, evidence and theories.
- Taking a distanced, critical stance towards subject matter, assumptions and explanations.
- Tackling issues systematically, logically and effectively.
- Examining the adequacy of evidence and checking alternative interpretations of it.
- Demonstrating a thorough understanding of complex, abstract concepts within the discipline.
- Writing clearly and cogently, following appropriate academic styles and conventions.
- Being able to set and solve problems by applying concepts and techniques appropriately.

However, in university-based healthcare courses, aims of higher education are assessed mostly in theoretical assessments, where critical analysis, problem solving, and evidence of arguments presented are expected.

As for Satterly's (1981) reference to assessments as invasions of privacy of the individual, this could apply to assessment of learners in that if a learner is struggling to achieve their practice competencies for no obvious reasons, then the mentor and others may probe for personal reasons for the learner not achieving. With an increasingly mature student population, family responsibilities, single motherhood, and having to hold down part-time jobs while on the pre-registration course could all well be reasons for a student not being able to give course matters sufficient attention, and therefore not achieving. Some students can be put off by this and even drop out of the course for a better-paid vocation. Others may accept extra help.

It is also suggested that patient privacy could be invaded during assessments, in that instead of one healthcare professional performing a procedure with a patient, when student assessment is being conducted then the student and the mentor are both present. Students might also take longer to perform the procedure, and if the mentor asks the student questions during the assessment, then the procedure can be even more prolonged, with even the patient's body part being exposed for longer periods of time. Additionally, in healthcare, invasion of privacy in assessment might also include problems of confidentiality, (e.g. in reflective write-ups in patient-based assessments).

Other problems with assessments have been identified by Rowntree (1987), Nicklin and Kenworthy (2000), Lankshear (1990) and Duffy (2004). Rowntree discusses some of the 'side-effects of assessments', referring to concepts such as self-fulfilling prophecy, whereby students who are expected to achieve low grades tend to achieve low grades, which might not necessarily be a reflection of the limitations of their innate ability. On the other hand, Nicklin and Kenworthy argue that the criticisms of assessments are essentially criticisms of inappropriately designed schemes of assessment in the curriculum, or faulty implementation. The findings of Lankshear's and Duffy's studies are discussed shortly.

## Difficulties with assessment of clinical skills

### Activity 7.4 – Difficulties with student assessment

Think about current day-to-day potential problems of assessments, and, considering them in the context of your own current place of work, first identify at least one clinical assessor who has already conducted quite a few clinical assessments. She or he does not need to be based solely in your workplace but should work broadly within your specialism. Your task is then to approach the assessor and ask them to explain precisely what steps they take in preparation for and in actually conducting assessment of competence with learners. Find out also from the assessor how they anticipate potential problems and avert them. Ask about some of the actual problems encountered, and the options they had for resolving them.

At the same time or afterwards, reflect for yourself on such problems and decide how you would go about dealing with them if they occurred in your own clinical setting.

*(Continued)*

Alternatively, think for yourself of all the problems that you might encounter in your assessment function as a mentor, and then the options that are available to you to resolve each of them.

Problems of assessment include differences in the interpretation of the exact meaning of placement objectives. There might be problems in conveying depth of knowledge expected, or level of skill demonstration. Issues like these can be rectified by open discussion between all personnel directly involved.

## Resolving problems of assessments

### Activity 7.5 – Resolving difficulties encountered by mentors

Refer back to Box 7.4 and work on the difficulties faced by mentors by identifying a number of problems of assessment you could encounter with a particular group of students, and the probable solutions for each of them. This can be done by completing Table 7.1.

The chances are you will be aware of or have thought of yet other problematic areas encountered by mentors in the assessment of learners, for which similar steps can be taken. They might include passing a student because the mentor likes the student, or failing because they dislike them, unqualified mentors signing up clinical competencies or misinterpretation of wording of practice competencies.

With some of these problem areas there could be instances when a mentor passes a student on a particular competency when they should be awarding a fail. This cannot be condoned, but failure to fail students has already been identified by Lankshear (1990), Duffy (2004) and others. If a student is failing, the mentor's professional judgement comes into play, and action plans are constructed.

*Action planning*
A mid-placement interview during the practice placement is an important component of assessment of students' progress with their placement competencies. The competencies will have been agreed at the beginning of the placement, and might be in the form of a learning contract. The mid-placement interview is technically a formal formative assessment point, which involves dedicated time for a discussion on the student's progress with placement competencies.

If the student has been progressing mostly as expected, then these are documented and the student continues as agreed in the learning contract. If the student has not been achieving as expected in either knowledge, skills and attitudes components, then an action plan needs to be constructed, which both mentor and learner mutually agree and sign. A practice educator or an academic such as the link tutor might

**Table 7.1 Criticisms or difficulties with assessments, and actions that can be taken to resolve them**

| Criticisms/difficulties with assessments | Actions that can be taken to resolve them |
| --- | --- |
| Leaving things to the last minute | |
| Difficulty with integration or ineffective application of theory and practice | |
| Personality problems/clashes | |
| Problems of organisation | |
| Lack of time for conducting assessments | |
| Student disagrees with mentor | |
| Attitude problems – student's or mentor's | |
| The service user or patient not consenting to student assessment | |
| Lack of resources (e.g. equipment) | |
| Structure of learning programme: variation of experience (e.g. allocation too short) | |
| (Other) | |

also be present and sign the action plan accordingly. An example of important components of an action plan is presented in Table 7.2 – it is usually laid out in landscape format.

Action planning involves specifying all components identified at the top of the table. If such an action plan was not constituted, then the student could have grounds for complaint and appeal if he or she is subsequently deemed a 'fail' for the placement. This point also indicates the importance of documentation of progress with achievement of placement objectives.

While there are some similarities between learning contracts and action plans, there are distinct differences between them in that the former is more learning centred, and the latter is more assessment centred. The learning contract is a systematic but speculative plan of learning based on practice competencies to be achieved and projected learning opportunities, and they may be adjusted during mid-placement progress discussions. The action plan is a 'must-achieve' device that identifies competencies that need to be achieved by an identified date during the practice placement, non-achievement of which would lead to a 'fail' mark being awarded.

*Reassessing the learner*
Once the action plan has been agreed, it must be adhered to, in that the mentor (or practice educator) and the student jointly ensure that the competencies are being

**Table 7.2  Example of an action plan**

| ACTION PLAN | | Mentee's name: | | Mentor's name: | | |
|---|---|---|---|---|---|---|
| Mentee's learning needs | Specific objectives to be achieved | Who will help mentee achieve the objectives and how? | Other resources required | Achieve by dates | Evidence of achievement of objectives |
| | | | | | |
| | | | | | |
| | | | | | |
| | | | | | |
| | | | | | |
| **AGREEMENT OF ACTION PLAN** | | | | | | |
| Mentor's signature: .............  Date: ........  Student's signature: ...........  Date: ........ | | | | | | |
| **ACHIEVEMENT OF OBJECTIVES** | | | | | | |
| Mentor's signature: .............  Date: ........ | | | | | | |

acquired, continuous assessment is occurring and, when ready, the student is reassessed and the documentation signed as and when achieved. The action plan is regularly reviewed and at the agreed date a final review is conducted.

The components discussed in this section address mostly the duties of the mentor. The next section considers the ethical and legal aspects of mentoring.

## Ethical and Legal Aspects of Assessments

All registrants have to comply with their professional body's code of conduct or practice, and this applies to mentoring or supervising juniors' and colleagues' learning as well. 'Professional and ethical practice' is one of the 'domains' of proficiency (along with related outcomes) that the NMC (2004b) identifies as components that the student nurse must achieve for gaining entry to the professional register. Therefore the mentor should already be competent in this component of professional practice through their pre-registration preparation, while their mentees will be developing these through theirs. On exploring the ethics of mentoring, Brown (2005) suggests that the mentor needs to be aware of their own values and ethical interpretations of clinical practice to enable mentees to develop 'ethical competence'.

Ethics refers to the social behaviours, morals and values of individuals and groups in relation to doing good for the greatest number, and to the impact or end results of clinical interventions (adapted from Brown, 2005). One widely accepted set of principles of ethics that apply to many spheres of life including medicine, business and education has been formulated by Thiroux and Krasemann (2007). These principles are:

- the value of life;
- goodness and rightness;
- justice and fairness;
- truth-telling and honesty;
- individual freedom.

These principles apply directly to mentoring in the following way:

- *The value of life* – can refer to ensuring mentees develop the necessary competencies for effective clinical interventions that would restore health and well-being. It can also refer to ensuring mentees acquire the necessary knowledge, skills and attitudes to register as a nurse so that they can earn a livelihood.
- *Goodness and rightness* – refer to the mentor doing good to mentees and patients or service users, and doing the right things.
- *Justice and fairness* – refer to ensuring that knowledge, skills and attitudes are acquired by all mentees to the appropriate extent, depth and detail.
- *Truth-telling and honesty* – ensuring incorrect information is not given.
- *Individual freedom* – means that mentees have some freedom in deciding the amount and type of learning, and patients or service users have some say in the clinical interventions available.

Other principles of ethics include (a) autonomy; (b) beneficence (doing good); and (c) non-maleficence (doing no harm). Furthermore, the British Association for Counselling and Psychotherapy's (2006) 'ethical framework' for counselling encompass values, principles and personal moral qualities. Values refer to respecting human rights and dignity, alleviating personal distress and suffering, and fairness. Personal moral qualities include empathy, sincerity, humility and competence.

Gallagher and Wainwright (2005), reporting on deliberations at the annual RCN Congress, however, indicate that much of nursing ethics are theoretical level academic discourses and do not translate into day-to-day practice and eventualities regularly encountered by healthcare professionals. They suggest that ethics is subjective, and competent ethical practice depends to a good extent on the integrity, honesty and moral behaviour of the healthcare professional.

---

☀️💡 **Think Point 7.3 – Application of principles of ethics**

Think of healthcare professionals whom you know personally, and consider in some detail how far you agree with Gallagher and Wainwright's (2005) suggestions that ethics is much talk and less application. Consider this also in the context of Thiroux and Krasemann's (2007) principles of ethics.

---

The codes of practice of healthcare professional regulatory bodies often incorporate ethical principles that registrants have to follow. As for mentors' relevant ethical practice in the assessment of competence, they should for instance not award a pass to a student for any particular competency if they are not completely sure that the latter can perform the clinical intervention competently.

The NMC (2006a) standards for mentors emphasise effective mentoring practices through the competences and outcomes for mentoring it has identified. For instance, under the domain 'Assessment and accountability', it specifies that the mentor must be competent to 'manage failing students so that they may enhance their performance and capabilities for safe and effective practice' (2006: 50). This competence implicitly suggests that mentoring practices must also comply with ethical and legal aspects of both patient or service user safety and care, and of facilitation of learning and assessment of learners' competence.

Furthermore, Duffin (2005) notes that mentors could face misconduct proceedings if they pass students who are incompetent, and that the NMC indicates that they will try to support mentors who feel unsupported if they wanted to fail students. This is because it seems that in the past some mentors felt they would not be given this support. Giving mentors 'protected time' for mentoring is also again advocated.

One of the legal implications of assessments is that on being awarded a pass, the individual is being given a licence and the legal right to practise the skill unsupervised when they register with their professional body. Awarding a licence to practise to someone who is not competent is technically in breach of the law. The clauses of the NMC (2004a) *COPC* clearly indicate that all registrants (i.e. including healthcare mentors) are personally accountable and answerable for their practice and must 'adhere to the laws of the country'.

A feature that frequently surfaces when the legality of the actions of registrants is questioned is the documentation of the actions taken. The NMC (2005a) and various other authorities clearly indicate that if an action is not recorded then it cannot be seen as having been done. For instance, Kendall-Raynor (2007) reports on the case of a registered nurse who had allegedly failed to supervise a mentee adequately, which resulted in the wrong dose of medication being given to a patient, who subsequently died. The case was dropped by the Crown Prosecution Service 'because of insufficient evidence', although it was due to be heard by the NMC's conduct and competence committee in 2007. This is an example of when legal and ethical aspects of mentoring may reflect different perspectives.

All four professional bodies directly involved in healthcare, namely the HPC, NMC, General Medical Council and General Social Care Council, either explicitly or implicitly incorporate such ethical components as respect of patient or service user as individuals, obtaining consent prior to clinical interventions, protecting confidential information, and identifying and minimising risk to patients or service users through their codes of practice.

Translating the principles of ethics into current healthcare practice addressing accountability, informed consent, confidentiality (including record keeping), professional misconduct, delegation and supervision.

## Responsibility and accountability of the mentor

All healthcare professionals are accountable for delivering care competently (NMC, 2004a), and also for other components of their roles such as enabling healthcare learners and colleagues develop their clinical skills. We are accountable to our patients, ourselves, our employers, our professional regulatory bodies, and in fact also to the general public.

To be responsible implies being answerable for one's actions, and it is a component of accountability. However, Stuart (2007) notes that before the registrant can be accountable, certain preconditions have to prevail, namely (a) the ability (knowledge, skills and attitude) to decide and act on a specific issue; (b) responsibility; and (c) authority.

One of the main thrusts of the mentor's accountability is related to the rules, regulations, policies and scope of practice that govern assessments. These are usually detailed in the appropriate mentor's handbook issued by the associated HEI, and briefly in the student's practice competencies or outcomes booklet for the placement. It is also related to specific eventualities in the assessment of professional competence, to implementation of assessment strategies, to personal and professional responsibilities, and to the relevant legislation. You would need to refer to the mentee's placement competencies booklet and to your professional regulatory body's code of practice for further clarification when needed.

The healthcare professional's mentoring responsibilities direct the spotlight on one specific area of their several professional roles, that of developing and improving the professional expertise of their mentees.

### Activity 7.6 – Teaching and learning as components of professional conduct

Refer to your professional regulatory body's code of practice and the partner HEI's guidelines on mentoring for your own profession, and ascertain how they express your responsibilities in terms of teaching (and assessing) others.

You will have noticed that a few clauses in the codes of practice directly identify registrants' teaching and own CPD responsibilities and roles. This is usually also a component of healthcare professionals' job description (or contract of employment) for the post they occupy.

Registrants may not transfer or delegate their accountability to another person. The mentor also functions under legal obligations for knowing about the mentee's course curriculum and built-in assessment procedures and regulations set out by the relevant HEI, and the appeals system that the mentee needs to follow if they feel they are being unjustly treated (Open University, 2001). Students have a right to appeal against the conduct of the assessment, but not against the mentor's decision to pass or fail, or their professional judgement about safe practice.

In accepting the role of mentor, the registrant is implicitly accepting responsibility and accountability for maintaining standards of supervision and assessment. The mentor's accountability for student learning is not fully clear, and instances of concern are investigated in their own right. However, the mentor must ensure that students gain the necessary clinical experiences to develop their professional competence and that the mentee does 'no harm' to the patient or service user, by teaching them the correct way of performing clinical procedures.

Rowntree (1987) indicates that there are times when the mentor might intentionally give permission to the learner to perform clinical interventions while supervising them unobtrusively, which can be expected, but at the same time assessing their performance without having specified this to them beforehand. This is sometimes referred to as 'hidden assessment', and could be another instance of unethical action by the mentor.

Furthermore, both initial preparation and continuing development are the joint responsibility of healthcare trusts and HEIs. Making professional judgements about the performance of students, and their ability to provide professionally competent and safe care, constitutes an endeavour to achieve predictive validity and reliability.

The NMC (2004a) *COPC* states that the interests of the patient or service user are paramount, that is, accountability to the patient or service user is more important than accountability to the student. However, the legal perspective can be, depending on individual situations, that the student is also answerable for incompetent interventions. Lack of experience or knowledge is not an acceptable reason for incompetent care.

On not being awarded a pass for a skill that was not performed competently, the learner might feel either merely disappointed or emotionally distraught. The mentor then needs to contact the practice educator or link tutor that further help and support might be needed, but might also have to use basic counselling skills (Quinn and Hughes, 2007) to help the learner. As for all professional skills, if the mentor does not feel able to perform these skills competently, then they should refer the learner to an appropriate professional who does have those skills.

## Supporting the Struggling or Underachieving Student

The mentor's leadership includes careful planning of practice placement to ensure practice objectives are achieved. However, it is well appreciated that, for a number of reasons, some student could be seen as struggling or even failing to show consistent learning and progress during the placement. So what are the different reasons for a student failing to achieve as expected?

---

**Think Point 7.3 – The struggling student**

From your own experience of students who struggle to achieve their clinical competencies, think of the different reasons for this happening during clinical placements.

---

Some students genuinely experience obstacles that intervene in their achievement of placement objectives. Could this be because they are working extra shifts to supplement their income, and therefore are not able to find sufficient time to work on their practice objectives? There can be several reasons. The RCN (2005a) suggests that if a student is not achieving the necessary competencies, then the mentor should take the following actions:

- Meet with the student as soon as possible to discuss this issue, and ensure the student knows the reason for the meeting.
- Inform the HEI contact person, associate mentor and clinical placement/practice facilitator so that both you (the mentor) and the student have independent support available.
- Clarify the area of weakness and advise how to progress.
- Form a realistic action plan to address the issues, and set deadlines.
- Work closely with the student.
- Arrange for the student to work with other assessors to ensure fairness.
- Make provision for any extra support or opportunities to improve within the practice area that the student may require.
- Keep careful notes of all discussions and incidents.

Individual HEIs tend to provide their own specific guidelines on the actions to take to support the struggling student.

---

## Activity 7.7 – Failing to fail students

So for one reason or another, a student might not be progressing as expected, and the mentor is not convinced that particular competencies will be achieved. However, on occasion mentors still decide to pass the student, as found by Duffy (2004).

Consider the whole spectrum of reasons why you think a mentor might award a pass to a student for a particular competency, even if the student has not demonstrated competent performance. List as many reasons as you can think of.

You should have been able to think of various day-to-day circumstances that might lead to the mentor awarding a pass to a failing student, none of which is a justifiable reason. These could include for instance pressure from the student, who ndicates that it is the last week of placement and that they have passed all previous placement competencies so far, and insufficient time allocated for assessing competencies.

## Case Study – The failing student

Bina is a pre-registration student on an eight-week placement at the end of her CFP. Her mentor has varied roles as part of their managerial functions, and has to cover extra shifts on days and nights due to staff sickness. However, Bina's placement has been marked by her frequent absence from the clinical setting due to sickness, and occasional tearfulness, claiming to feel depressed. She has been advised to seek help from the trust's Occupational Health Department, and has been made aware that she can access the university's counselling facility if preferred.

Shortly after the placement started, the practice educator went on maternity leave, and it took a few weeks to install a replacement for her. The acting practice educator contacted Bina's personal tutor to explain Bina's circumstances and was advised that, among other things, a mid-placement interview needed to be conducted to ascertain Bina's progress with practice competencies, and documented accordingly. In particular, if these competencies were not achieved, then Bina would fail the CFP and not progress to the adult branch programme. The student is described as lacking in motivation and as 'a real struggle' by the acting practice educator.

Due to Bina's continuing absence and health problem, the mid-placement interview only took place quite late in the placement, and an action plan was instituted as various practice competencies had still not been achieved.

Consider what would be the specialist helping or counselling skills that could be utilised in regular mentor–mentee contact if both Bina and her mentor were more available.

As indicated earlier, 'failure to fail' has been identified as a dilemma over a number of years (e.g. Duffy, 2004; Lankshear, 1990). At times the mentor may have done all the planning for the student to achieve competencies, and yet on assessment they might find that the student has not reached the level of competence required to award them a pass for particular competencies. This could mean failing the practice placement. Consequently, the student's placement may have to be extended to allow them more time to achieve the competencies, and their course extended. Some students are likely to become upset or ashamed at failing the placement, or maybe they did all they could but still did not achieve. The mentor will then need to draw on their helping skills to help the student further.

## Helping and counselling the struggling student

The general and specific communication skills needed to establish a relationship and support the mentee develop and achieve competencies were explored to some extent in Chapter 1. In particular, the 'Communication continuum – related skills, and who uses them' detailed by Scammell (1990) (see Table 1.1) suggests that specific communication skills are needed for helping students who are struggling to achieve their clinical competencies, or who may be struggling with the nursing course as a whole and are even in danger of failing in their chosen career.

It is suggested at this point that you refresh your understanding of the communication skills discussed in Chapter 1. In addition to the generic communication skills that are necessary for all effective relationships, specialist communication skills are also required by the mentor to deal with more problematic situations.

The special skill of 'counselling' is one of the roles of the teacher (Quinn and Hughes, 2007), and increasingly that of the mentor for the reasons just discussed. First, however it is well recognised that for counselling to be effective the process should be entered into voluntarily by the person being counselled (the counsellee). Indeed it is generally agreed that unless counselling is actively sought by the counsellee, the interaction might not be as effective, even if the helper uses most of the skills used in counselling. Second, counselling is a therapeutic technique requiring specialist training. Persons not skilled in its use will, at best, not help the counsellee, and at worst potentially compound the counsellee's problems. Therefore, unless they are fully qualified as counsellors, mentors and other teachers in healthcare are more likely to use helping or 'basic' counselling skills. For more intense mentee problems, referral should be made to specialist services such as the university's counselling service, which is usually a section of student services provision.

The most important factor within a counselling situation is the relationship between the counsellor and the counsellee. This was identified initially by Rogers (1983) and later by Rogers and Freiberg (1994), both identifying three key qualities (also known as 'core conditions' of helping) that are required for effective counselling. These key qualities, as detailed under student-centred teaching in Chapter 3, are genuineness, trust and acceptance and empathic understanding.

In addition to the generic communication skills, verbal and non-verbal, the key helping skills identified by Quinn and Hughes (2007) are self-awareness, attending, active listening, summarizing, reflecting, questioning, use of silence, and 'concreting'. This set of skills can be used as a framework for checking how thoroughly you feel you dealt with these situations. By analysing your interactions with others you will develop a greater awareness of how far you as a professional are able to help others.

Dedicated time is required for a systematic approach to counselling. This is done by utilising a model of helping such as Heron's (1989) six-category intervention analysis. This model indicates six possible interactions between the two parties as detailed in Box 7.7. Alternatively, Berne's 'transactional analysis' approach can be implemented.

In the aforementioned case study, for instance, the mentor can help Bina by utilising components of Heron's framework. Instances of responses by the mentor to the student's account of his or her perception of the situation are as follows:

- *Prescriptive* – advise Bina to reduce less important life activities to concentrate on working to achieve her placement objectives as a priority.
- *Informative* – give information on professional and personal matters as appropriate (e.g. location of Occupational Health Department).
- *Confrontational* – ask Bina directly what she is doing or how she could behave differently for a more amiable experience.
- *Supportive* – allow Bina time and silence to think over the mentor's questions and suggestions.
- *Cathartic* – allow Bina to verbalise in ample detail why she is struggling in this placement.
- *Catalytic* – the mentor acts as facilitator to enable Bina to meet her learning needs.

## Activity 7.9 – A struggling student you have encountered

Think of a student whom you have known to have failed to achieve required practice objectives resulting in to the student being disappointed, upset or distressed. In case you haven't encountered such a student, think of a situation that you might encounter. Describe the situation in up to 75 words. Then, utilising Heron's (1989) six-category intervention analysis framework, identify the specific actions that you could take, using each of the categories to help the student.

Alternatively consider Mel Alexis's situation cited in Chapter 1, and follow the above instructions.

Hawkins and Shohet (2006) suggest taking an inter-subjective approach that focuses on the relationship between mentor and mentee. This notion largely implies using empathy. Universities usually provide a counselling service for any student who is distressed about any issue that is affecting their progress with their course. To become a skilled counsellor especially for dealing with particular psychological problems requires several years of structured educational preparation. However, Hawkins and Shohet also provide a number of pointers on how supervisors can help, such as by developing 'the qualities of a good supervisor' in themselves, which are noted in Box 7.5.

---

### Box 7.5   Qualities of a good supervisor

- Flexibility with use of different concepts and intervention methods
- A multi-perspective view (i.e. being able to see the situation from different angles)
- A working map of the discipline or subject area
- The ability to work transculturally
- The ability to contain or manage anxiety of self and supervisee, or refer to an appropriate agency
- Openness to learning from supervision situations
- Sensitivity to the impact of wider contextual issues on the supervision process
- Awareness of different types of power and how to handle them
- Humour, humility and patience

*Source:* adapted from Hawkins and Shohet (2006).

---

Proctor's (2001) 'supervision alliance model' is widely accepted as a suitable framework for systematic supervision. As a model of helping that is also acknowledged by Hawkins and Shohet, it comprises three main functions or roles of the helper, namely normative, formative and restorative.

Although the mentor is expected to exercise professional judgement and make pass or fail decisions on particular student performances, there are support networks that they can draw on whenever unsure. Informal or formal team mentoring and peer consultation frameworks might already be in place, but, as indicated in this chapter, the mentor's copy of practice competencies booklets normally contains full details regarding the procedure to follow in these circumstances, such as contacting the practice educator.

This chapter has explored ways in which the mentor exercises leadership. However, it is useful to note that the leadership role is not just about taking actions to avert problems. It is also about taking action to achieve aims and good practice. Sines et al. (2006) report on joint actions taken by an NHS trust and the partner university to ensure student nurses achieve fitness for practice by the end of the three-year pre-registration course. Most of the mechanisms instituted are not unknown, but several of them were planned in substantial detail. These mechanisms include:

- identifying core skill clusters;
- adapted OSCEs;
- enhanced clinical skills laboratories;
- an additional training programme in assessment of skills for existing mentors;
- regular mentoring updates;
- appointment of practice educators.

## Chapter Summary

This chapter has focused on leadership and the challenges of mentoring, particularly in relation to assessments and, having completed this chapter, you will have learned about:

- The mentor's leadership in careful forward planning of assessments, making decisions and giving feedback to the student after assessing them perform clinical skills. Good practice guidelines for assessments.
- Current criticisms of, and difficulties with, assessment of clinical skills, followed by how these problems are averted.
- Actual or potential problems of assessment of competencies, resolving these problems, including action planning and reassessment of the learner.
- The responsibility and accountability of the mentor in ensuring that a pass or fail is awarded as appropriate, and relevant subsequent actions taken.
- Use of professional judgement, and how intra- and inter-mentor reliability can be monitored and achieved; and the ethical and legal aspects of mentoring.
- How underachieving or struggling students can be supported using basic communication and helping skills, and more specialist communication skills, including counselling. They constitute skills that would also apply to student assessment situations, and include time management and proactive actions, and the use of support networks with peers, practice educators and academic staff.

# EIGHT

# Evaluating Mentoring

## Introduction

This chapter addresses the evaluation role of the mentor, and covers:

- Why evaluate mentoring activities, focusing largely on the evaluation of facilitation of learning and assessment of competencies.
- Exactly what is evaluation, and who evaluates mentoring activities?
- How mentors evaluate learning provision in their clinical settings, use of models of evaluation, and how they evaluate assessments.
- The actions to take with the results of evaluations, the problems, consequences and opportunities.
- Continuing professional development for mentors based on available opportunities, and the mentor as a lifelong learner.

Evaluation of learning, which is one of the eight domains of mentoring activities identified by the NMC in *Standards for Supporting Learning and Assessment in Practice* (2006a), is examined in this chapter, the other seven domains having already been discussed in preceding chapters. Evaluation of mentoring therefore amounts to mentors self-monitoring the effectiveness and quality of their mentoring activities, and includes intra- and inter-mentor reliability in assessments, which was discussed in Chapter 7 as one of the likely challenges of mentoring. Evaluation information forms the basis for progressive learning, and therefore also the mentor's own continuing professional development.

## Chapter outcomes

On completion of the chapter you should be able to:

1. Give a number of reasons for evaluating facilitation of learning and assessment of competencies.
2. Explain the nature and various features of evaluation.
3. Identify different ways of evaluating clinically based and academically based teaching and assessment.
4. Justify the actions that should be taken following evaluations and the likely difficulties with this activity.
5. Explain how the challenges encountered by mentors also offer opportunities for professional development, and for ongoing learning.

## Why Evaluate Mentoring Activities?

The reason for evaluating mentoring activities is that it is logical to do so, either to confirm that mentoring practices are and remain effective, or to identify likely areas for improvement. Registrants engage in evaluation of care and treatment continually during any span of duty, and therefore it is not an unfamiliar activity to them. The specific competence and outcomes under the domain 'evaluation of learning' set by the NMC (2006a) for mentors are as follows:

- *Competence for 'evaluation of learning' domain* – determine strategies for evaluating learning in practice and academic settings to ensure that the NMC's standards of proficiency for registration or recording a qualification at a level above initial registration have been met.
- *Outcomes* – (a) contribute to evaluation of student learning and assessment experiences, proposing aspects for change resulting from such evaluation, and (b) participate in self- and peer evaluation to facilitate personal development and contribute to the development of others.

The 'NMC standards of proficiency' were discussed in some detail in Chapters 2 and 6 in the context of 'what' healthcare students need to learn, and be assessed on, respectively. Self- and peer evaluation were also discussed to some extent in Chapter 6.

## Activity 8.1 – Why evaluate?

Consider the question why we should evaluate anyway, and what we can do with information gathered from evaluations, and make some notes.

There are a number of reasons for evaluation. If mentors do not evaluate their mentoring activities, then they are taking for granted that their actions meet their learners' learning needs. They are assuming that learners are satisfied with the learning provided, and that they are fulfilling their roles effectively. Formal evaluations often reveal unexpected impressions, and therefore the reality might be different. Further reasons for evaluation are:

- To identify improvement points for subsequent mentoring activities.
- To gauge whether the mentee's learning is pitched at the appropriate level.
- Continuing self-assessment of competence in professional practice is often a requirement of employment.
- It is a component of the clinical setting's quality assurance mechanism.
- It is professional 'good practice'.

Just as in any problem-solving approach which tends to entail assessment, planning, implementation and evaluation, systematic approaches to most novel ventures entail evaluation of the plans implemented and the actions to be taken subsequent to evaluation. If the mentor or teacher does not evaluate their teaching, then what evidence will they have of their effectiveness? Additionally, Rogers (2002) indicates that in education, we evaluate so as to:

- Improve our teaching.
- Plan new strategies and identify hindrances, and decide what to do about them.
- Ascertain how much progress has been made, and the direction and distance to go with our teaching.

## Activity 8.2 – Can evaluation of teaching improve learning?

Focusing on the mentor's teaching role, consider the evaluation of teaching that you have experienced, and identify at least two ways in which this can lead to improvement in learning.

Healthcare course lecturers are required to evaluate their teaching and act on the evaluation data. Furthermore, as for the evaluation tool used, the NMC recognises that such tools need to be 'fit for purpose', rather than just convenient tools that might be inappropriate for the job. 'Fit for purpose' means exactly what the term states, that is, the tool has to be appropriate for achieving the objectives of the setting or organisation, and should meet the quality criteria of a quality assurance model. Following evaluation of teaching, the mentor can follow the teaching component up with further articles or information to help students meet their learning needs. They can arrange further teaching sessions on topics suggested in the evaluation information, and can also adjust their subsequent teaching with a view to further improvement.

## What is Evaluation?

Most health professionals are familiar with the concept of evaluation of care, as it constitutes a key component of a systematic approach to care and treatment, and is an inherent facet of care pathways.

## Activity 8.3 – What does the term evaluation itself mean?

Make brief notes on what you understand by the word evaluation. What is it about?

Evaluation of the effectiveness of care given is important. Evaluation is also an essential facet of professional education programmes in healthcare in order to review or ascertain how effectively and efficiently the curriculum meets the stated philosophy, aims and objectives of the course. It is a part of the process that reviews the currency and value of the original aims and philosophy of a course or module.

The term *evaluation* originates from the French word *evaluer*, meaning to work out the numerical value of something. In current usage in English it means appraising or making a judgement about the worth of something (Brown, 2002: 871). Various definitions of evaluation have been offered by interested parties over the years. For instance, Roberts et al. (2001) indicate that evaluation is essentially about making judgements about the value and worth of something against explicit, justifiable and appropriate criteria. Thus evaluation is the process of systematically collecting and analysing information in order to form value judgements based on firm evidence. An exploration of evaluation therefore comprises:

- Precisely what is to be evaluated and how?
- Who should be involved?
- How to evaluate?
- What to do with the evaluation data?

---

 ### Think Point 8.1 – What do we evaluate?

When evaluating care in clinical practice, exactly what is it that we evaluate, and what are the different ways in which evaluation information is obtained?

---

Broadly speaking, evaluation data can be obtained by:

- Direct observation of general state or appearance of a patient or situation.
- Monitoring whether instructions are being followed.
- Measurements and pathology laboratory results.
- Casual conversation.
- Asking the patient.
- Using questionnaires.

Other terms that tend to have similar or overlapping meanings with evaluation are assessment, quality appraisal and monitoring. However, assessment has a distinct and specific meaning in healthcare, referring to assessment of patients' health problems, and of learners' competence. Rogers (2002) distinguishes between assessment and evaluation by suggesting that assessment refers to the collection of data against set criteria. It is therefore objective. Evaluation refers to the values and personal judgement of the recipient of the activity.

However, evaluation is also used as an empirical tool in the form of a research method involving in-depth exploration of the component being evaluated through data collection and analysis. In Guba and Lincoln's (1989) fourth-generation evaluation as a research method, the first-generation evaluation is measurement orientated, the second generation is based on measurable objectives, the third generation is judgement orientated, and the fourth generation in based on negotiation. These concepts can be seen as models of evaluation. Redfern (1998) refers to other models of evaluation such as pragmatic evaluation (which begins by ascertaining the practical value of the component), pluralist evaluation (combining several models to form a new one), and realistic model of evaluation (exploring the mechanics of explanation). These concepts may appear almost esoteric to the mentor, but then they do belong to arenas of highly skilled and stringent empirical activities.

Returning to evaluation of mentoring, this can also be public or private, external or internal, continuous or episodic/intermittent and final (refers to time scale). Moreover, evaluation can be case-specific or generalised/holistic or analytical (see Box 8.1 for a brief explanation of these).

---

**Box 8.1  Who evaluates what?**

| | |
|---|---|
| *Public evaluation* | Open evaluation of an activity by others |
| *Private evaluation* | Self-evaluation by the person who performed the teaching, for instance |
| *External evaluation* | Evaluation by others outside the organisation |
| *Internal evaluation* | Evaluation by departments or individuals inside the organisation |
| *Continuous evaluation* | Ongoing evaluation |
| *Episodic/intermittent evaluation* | Evaluation at set or specific times |
| *Final evaluation* | Evaluation at the end of one or a series of activities |
| *Case-specific evaluation* | In-depth evaluation of one particular instance of an activity |
| *Generalised or holistic evaluation* | Inviting and gaining overall impressions |
| *Analytical evaluation* | Detailed evaluation, may include numerical data |

---

Neary (2000a) adds that evaluation can be quantitative or qualitative. Generally for new topic areas, qualitative evaluation is likely to elicit data that can enable further development of the topic. For more established topic areas, quantitative data are sought to monitor or ascertain the likely ongoing effectiveness of the activity.

The evaluation of patient or service user care and of teaching episodes is undertaken formatively and summatively. Formative evaluation of care is a continuous activity, the frequency of which is adjusted according to the dependency level of the patient/service user, or to the criticality of their condition. With some service users who require longer-term care, or those in the community, evaluation may be recorded at longer intervals at specific set periods. Summative evaluations are conducted at end points, for example of a care pathway, or a specific part of it.

Evaluation is also one of the four stages of the development review process of healthcare professionals identified in the *NHS KSF* (DoH, 2004b). The first stage is the joint review of the individual's work against the demands of the post. This is in the context of the six core dimensions of healthcare work. The second is the personal development planning stage, the third is the learning and development stage, and the fourth is the evaluation stage. In the evaluation stage, the individual:

- Reflects on the effectiveness of their learning and development of their knowledge and skills.
- Identifies how their learning has improved the application of their learning to their post.
- Feeds back to the organisation on how the learning and development can be improved.

Furthermore, job evaluation is another related concept that is a feature of banding of healthcare professionals' posts under *Agenda for Change* (DoH, 2001a).

In the context of evaluating mentoring, this textbook focuses on all the above aspects of evaluation except evaluation as a research method. Having examined why we need to evaluate mentoring activities and exactly what evaluation is, it is also important to consider who evaluates before moving on to how mentors evaluate their mentoring.

## Who evaluates teaching and learning?

As mentioned earlier, evaluation can take different forms (see Box 8.2). Formative evaluation of teaching and learning is conducted through informal and formal mechanisms. It is a micro-level evaluation that the mentor performs informally when teaching clinical interventions, either in the clinical area or in university settings. It is a valuable internal mechanism for monitoring one's own competence through a continuous process of observation and sensory feedback.

There is also the formal evaluation mechanism that requires more concrete evidence to be gathered and reproduced when required. Formal evaluation mechanisms can manifest patterns of good or poor teaching delivery. These formal evaluation exercises take place periodically and allow scrutiny of the quality of theoretical and clinical learning. For instance, during the clinical placement, the student also engages in a continuous process of informal evaluation of the extent to which the clinical setting is also a learning environment.

---

**Think Point 8.2 – Evaluation of teaching in the clinical setting**

Who in your experience evaluates the effectiveness of teaching, both planned and informal or opportunistic, in the clinical area?

---

In general, it is the recipient of the teaching, that is, the learner, who is best placed to evaluate the effectiveness of the teaching. Additionally, the result of the teaching will also emerge in the knowledge and skill acquired by the learner and ultimately be reflected in the quality of patient or service user care. In addition to the mentor engaging in self-evaluation or self-monitoring the quality of their work-based teaching and assessment, however, in addition to self-evaluation, the quality of their work-based teaching and assessment can also be ascertained through peer evaluation. Furthermore, evaluation can also be conducted by individual professionals, by clinical teams, or at organisational level.

Generally, there are at least two parties interested in the quality of a service: the provider, and the consumer or user. It seems obvious to suggest that to ensure consumers get maximum quality from the service, the providers need first to find out what the consumer wants or needs, and then to be able to deliver the service required. The current purchaser–provider ethos has prevailed in healthcare since the NHS and Community Care Act (DoH, 1990). The consumers of mentoring activities are mentors' learners, and the university at which they are students, as well as patients or service users.

## Activity 8.4 – Who is interested in evaluation?

Think of all personnel and agencies that are likely to be interested in the effectiveness and quality of healthcare courses at universities, and jot down specifically who they are.

The quality of healthcare courses is of interest to both purchasers and consumers of the provision. Purchasers of education are generally students, many of whom pay their course fees themselves. For healthcare profession courses, the purchaser is the NHS trusts for most pre- and post-registration courses, and individual students based in the NHS or the independent sector (e.g. private hospitals and nursing or residential homes). Other NHS trusts may be regular purchasers of certain courses, as are healthcare students from overseas, and professionals who qualified overseas but are seeking professional registration in the UK. The quality of courses is also of interest to ward managers and other qualified colleagues directly dealing with students and who have certain expectations of them during and after the course, and also the public who expects expert professional care.

Strategic Health Authorities (SHAs), and Primary Care and NHS Trusts identify the broad areas of educational programmes required for healthcare staff to meet the clinical intervention and health needs of the local population. Within a climate of purchasers and providers, educational establishments have to market their educational services and provide evidence of quality assurance measurement within their contracts for services. Purchasers and consumers can also be seen as users of the service. However, as professional learning takes place in clinical as well as university settings, learning is a partnership agreement between trusts, education providers and students to enable effective delivery of expected professional education.

Other stakeholders interested in the quality of educational provision, as this ultimately impacts on patients or service users' health, are at organisational level, where evaluation is conducted through internal audit mechanisms, and externally by the QAA, the NMC, HPC and other regulatory bodies. Other universities who specialise in education in the subject being evaluated might also be involved. Evaluation by healthcare trusts occurs through feedback from NHS and Primary Care trusts regarding fitness for practice, evaluation of clinical placements, and mentors' feedback to the partner university. A number of ways of evaluating education programmes and the various agencies involved in evaluating learning, teaching and assessment are explored in the next section.

## How Mentors Evaluate Learning Provision

Having ascertained what evaluation is and who evaluates, this section explores how evaluation is conducted. The wide range of learners whose learning the mentor is likely to facilitate includes learners from different healthcare professions and those not following specific programmes of study, and can include patients and their relatives, as identified in Chapter 3.

Evaluation is not always a favoured exercise as, according to Handy (1989), highest-quality service is not easily achieved, since it needs the right equipment, the right people and the right environment, which might not always be fully available. It engenders opinions from all interested parties, who might also set new goals for changing educational provision. Quantitative and qualitative information is obtained through the use of structured or semi-structured forms with selected headings. Such information can also be obtained through verbal or written means.

### Activity 8.5 – Evaluating facilitation of learning

Think back to a teaching session you delivered recently. You may have taught a student, a colleague or a patient or service user, either a particular clinical skill or a component of knowledge. Which aspects did you feel you ought to evaluate to gain a measure of the effectiveness of the session? Furthermore, exactly how do we evaluate a formal teaching session? What are the methods available to the mentor?

Teachers are aware that one of the key elements of any teaching session or learning provision is its evaluation. The teaching and learning in the clinical setting session can be evaluated from a number of viewpoints or conducted in various ways. As an internal evaluation mechanism, the teacher (i.e. the mentor) in the clinical setting decides which evaluation tool or model is the most appropriate to gain the necessary information about how a teaching session was received. Some of these tools are identified in Box 8.2.

---

### Box 8.2   Methods of evaluation of teaching in the clinical setting

- General discussion at the end of the session
- Verbal feedback – requested/volunteered
- Verbal questions and answers
- Feedback from the university through link tutors or practice educators
- Feedback from colleagues or peers, witness statement
- Quiz – on paper/verbal
- Observing how other teachers teach the skill
- Self-evaluation/reflection
- Using questionnaire(s)
- Observing/monitoring clinical skill performance – direct and indirect
- Continuous monitoring of student's general clinical competence and motivation to learn
- Checking whether objectives are being met
- Reflection/reflective account
- A short multiple-choice-type test
- Discussing booklet of competencies
- Asking the student to teach others (e.g. a patient or junior staff)
- Service user feedback
- Using evaluation form(s)

---

## Evaluating learning using models of evaluation

There are several models of evaluation that individuals or organisations can use as frameworks for systematically evaluating the quality of learning provision. Maxwell's (1984) six elements or dimensions of quality, is one of them. The six dimensions are: accessibility, acceptability, and appropriateness (3 As), and efficiency, effectiveness and equity (3 Es). Healthcare course providers can develop their own criteria using Maxwell's model for formal evaluation of quality of learning by asking questions related to each of the six dimensions. The education provider that aims and claims to offer a quality service should meet all these criteria. Some manage to do so explicitly, while others may be at different stages of development.

Another framework is provided by Lang's (1976) model of quality assurance. This model emphasises the process through a problem-solving approach. Yet another is the popular Donabedian (1988) model of quality assurance using standard statements, and structure, process and outcome components (e.g. RCN, 1990). This model was also discussed in the context of practice development in Chapter 5, and the evaluator may choose to evaluate all three components, or only the process component, or outcome.

Mentors, nurse lecturers and other education facilitators can use the Donabedian model to evaluate their learning facilitation. University modules and courses are generally evaluated using items under standard headings such as teaching, assessment and feedback, academic support, organisation and management, resources, personal development, and any other comments.

## Evaluating professional healthcare courses

### Activity 8.6 – Evaluating academic programmes

Consider education provision as a public service provided by a particular university with which you are familiar. What criteria would you use to judge the quality of their programmes? Make a list of these criteria. Now try and identify issues or aspects that constitute good quality education provision, say in relation to a course you are interested in, in the health and social care department of the university.

If available, obtain local or national criteria that could be used to ascertain the quality of this service, say, from the Internet. Do they match your own criteria of quality, and do any of these standards match the services which are actually being provided?

The QAA conducts four-yearly audits of programmes offered by universities using their own evaluation framework, which are known as major reviews of healthcare programmes. The Department of Health, through a partnership comprising the NMC, the HPC and the SHAs, also carries out reviews of all NHS-funded healthcare programmes regularly. The QAA aims to provide public assurance that the quality and standards of higher education are being safeguarded and enhanced by conducting these reviews.

The areas that the QAA reviewers comment on are academic and practitioner standards, quality of learning opportunities (under learning and teaching), student progression, learning resources and their effective utilisation, maintenance and enhancement of standards and quality. Reviewers undertaking a major review look at:

- learning outcomes;
- the curriculum;
- student assessment;
- student achievement.

The reviewers then deliver one of the following judgements on academic and practitioner standards – 'confidence', 'limited confidence', or 'no confidence'. These 'subject review' headings can be used by universities for internal ongoing evaluation of programme provision. The QAA also publishes various guidelines documents which universities can use to gain an impression of the QAA's expectations.

The NMC on the other hand performs periodic review of programme provision using its own evaluation framework. Its latest venture is to develop a new *UK Wide Quality Assurance Framework* (NMC, 2006f). This comprises 20 standards, including institutional approval, programmes approval and reapproval, and the requirement for programme providers to submit an annual report to the NMC on all approved programmes.

A key component of these reviews (or audits) of university courses is that the reviewers' remits includes inspecting clinical settings where students gain clinical experience, and this can include interviewing mentors and clinical managers. Evaluation requires openness and trust by both parties, a willingness to be open about expectations, and about the strengths and weaknesses in the organisation. Appropriate resources are required to meet the specified standards and consumer expectations and needs.

In addition to Maxwell's, Lang's, Donabedian's, the QAA's and NMC's models or frameworks of evaluation, Dean (2000) refers to the classical evaluation model which specifically includes measurements of the extent to which the learning outcomes were achieved. However, evaluators normally seek quantitative as well as qualitative data by asking for further comments after each question. Furthermore, professional bodies such as the RCN (e.g. *Quality Education for Quality Care: A Position Statement for Nursing Education;* RCN, 2003]), the Royal College of Midwifery usually also recommend quality improvement measures on specific aspects of practice.

This chapter has so far examined the evaluation of teaching, learning provision and assessment. The next aspect to consider is the destination of the evaluation data.

As for module evaluation, the academic who is the module leader collects information about the module from students against particular criteria in relation to:

- Staff – whether they were well prepared, accessible, gave constructive feedback.
- Teaching and learning methods.
- Assessment – marking criteria, feedback.
- Resources – teaching rooms, library support, and online support.
- The module itself – its relevance, difficulty level, whether the module was well-organised, and achieved its aims and objectives.

The module leader has to present evaluation information at academic team meetings, together with the actions being taken to rectify any weaknesses identified, and should highlight other key issues. As stated before, the module itself will have undergone quality scrutiny prior to delivery to students. Assessment questions will have been peer reviewed, approved by the relevant internal committee and then by the external examiner. However, flaws in the delivery of the module may surface, due to, say, resource problems or with pass rates.

Usually, the module leader also has to report on the number of students who started on the course or module, how many completed on the first attempt, how many dropped out, and how many passed on resubmission. Internal moderators and external examiners report on quality of scripts, and consistency of marking is also considered.

Institutional evaluation issues are actioned or dealt with by heads of department or at Deanery level. Placement issues are jointly resolved by mentors and clinical managers, and university link tutors. Senior clinical managers and higher-level university personnel may be involved in resolving more major issues.

### Evaluating practice placements

Standards of teaching in practice settings are closely related to the quality of patient or service user care, the quality of student supervision, and the expertise of mentors. Students' learning experiences during placements are monitored jointly by the university and clinical managers. At the end of placements students are asked for feedback, often a written evaluation on various aspects such as whether they had adequate preparation for the placement, and given an orientation on the first day of placement.

On teaching and learning, students may be asked to comment on whether a named mentor had been identified, placement objectives were identified, the range of learning opportunities, feedback on performance of clinical skills, how often worked with a mentor, and whether evidence-based practice was prevalent. There could also be questions on the amount and nature of personal support available.

Evaluation information on the quality of the learning experience is imparted to the placement areas by the university. The mentor may have obtained qualitative evaluation information from the student prior to the end of the placement. Placement evaluations also form a basis for communication between professionals in clinical settings and university lecturers, and an additional benefit of the process is that training and development needs of clinical staff can be identified for both effective clinical care and for competent mentoring practice.

## Evaluation of assessments

The mentor performs numerous assessments of competencies in this role. How are the quality and efficacy of assessments performed by a mentor monitored? The mentor's professional judgement comes into play to some extent, as they have to be able to justify the decisions they make about the student's competence, in that the responsibility normally lies with the mentor to seek all information relevant to assessments, and to keep their own professional competence up to date. Furthermore, if a student feels the result of an assessment was unfair or incorrect, then he/she can appeal following appropriate procedures. This is usually only for the conduct of the assessment and any technical or practical interference during the assessment, but not against the professional judgement of the assessor.

Evaluation of assessment of theory is conducted through structured mechanisms. The pass mark for coursework or assignments for healthcare professional education courses is usually 40 per cent. Assignments are marked by module teams, final projects are double marked, and then a stratified sample of scripts is internally moderated, and then further scrutinised by external examiners. All are answerable to subject assessment boards and programme boards. Less clear student situations are debated, further advice is sought if necessary, and decisions are made using the university's rules and regulations and professional judgement.

---

 **Think Point 8.3 – Evaluating assessments**

Consider how the mentor evaluates the soundness of the assessments they perform. How do mentors ascertain that their own knowledge and competence in assessing students remain up to date, valid and reliable?

---

In response to Think Point 8.3 you may have felt that the mentor's accountability has a major role to play in ensuring that their own knowledge and competence in assessing students remain up to date, valid and reliable. This can be achieved by:

- Discussions on mentor update study days regarding, say, intra-mentor and inter-mentor reliability.
- Team mentoring (including assessing).
- Consulting link tutor, practice educator and/or senior colleague (e.g. ward sister).

Ways of achieving intra-mentor reliability were examined in Chapter 7.

## Evaluation Results and Development Opportunities

Rogers (2002) notes that accurate evaluation is one of the most difficult skills to acquire, especially if change is anticipated. It is also often an uncomfortable exercise as it may reveal unanticipated flaws, or perceived flaws depending on the evaluator's own state of mind and general outlook. There might be other biased views stated, or practical problems related to evaluation of teaching highlighted, whether the teaching be clinically based or classroom based.

Following on from these observations, this section explores problems and the possible consequences of evaluations, and their likely implications for CPD for mentors. Mentoring RNs on specialist practice courses, lifelong learning, support mechanisms for the mentor, and the use of professional development plans are also discussed.

### Problems and consequences of evaluations

As discussed throughout this book, the mentoring role of health professionals has various facets. Consequently, each facet involves a set of activities in itself, which requires relevant knowledge and competence. To ascertain how well each role is being performed, the mentor has to evaluate and self-monitor their performance, and also obtain feedback from mentees, peers and their own mentors or clinical supervisors. How much and how comprehensively does the mentor do this, and what do they do with the data obtained?

Mostly, this is not an issue because, as an accountable professional, the mentor continually endeavours to rectify any weakness in their performance and knowledge, and strives to enhance their practice at all times. However, there can be problems with evaluation of mentoring.

 **Think Point 8.4 – Issues with evaluation**

What do you feel are the likely problems associated with evaluation of the mentoring role?

A possible problem area or danger related to the evaluation of a teaching session is that the criticisms of one's earlier teaching sessions may give the impression that you are not quite cut out for teaching. However, teaching is one of the competencies of all qualified nurses and, like many other skills, can be learned and subsequently mastered with sufficient practice. It is also usually one of the items in the RN's job description. On self-evaluation of their mentoring functions (referred to by Rogers, 2002 as post-hoc evaluation), they may encounter weaknesses that they may not wish to reveal to others and choose to rectify them by trial and error.

Practice placement evaluations could also highlight serious problems with mentoring, as found by Phillips et al. (2000) for instance, that might not prove easy to resolve. The mentor needs to be able to differentiate between progress and levels of attainment by learners, as suggested by Rogers (2002). All learners may be making progress but they could be achieving at different levels depending on their educational background, efforts and time for study, and learning opportunities. Some of the likely problems of evaluation are as follows:

- Judgement aimed at influencing peers' opinions.
- Just one incident may colour statement about the whole session.
- Teacher may be a perfectionist and may feel very disappointed if weaknesses are pointed out.
- Points identified by students might not be seen as positive statements.
- May be seen as 'some you win, some you lose', and any action to work on suggested weaknesses might not be taken.
- The person might genuinely not appreciate the weaknesses pointed out.
- Difficult to be entirely objective.

Research and ensuing recommendations have highlighted problematic areas of mentoring practice and aspects that need developing. For instance, Philips et al. (2000) identified the role conflict that mentors encounter. Many of the challenges the mentor encounters are related to assessment of practice objectives, and are predominantly due to insufficient time because of having to fulfil their various roles. Many of these issues were identified in particular in Chapter 7 (in Box 7.4).

Furthermore, Duffy (2004) found that a problem previously identified by Lankshear (1990) more than a decade earlier – that is, mentors failing to fail incompetent students – was still prevalent. The NMC (2006a) responded by issuing new standards for mentors and other guidelines (e.g. NMC, 2006d), which may present as further professional development requirements for previously qualified mentors.

Duffin (2005) reports that the NMC remains concerned about the range of clinical expertise in the armoury of the newly qualified nurse, midwife or SCPHN. The NMC is therefore considering relaxing the rules on 'skills labs', in which students carry out simulated procedures on dummies. Such laboratories have almost always been in use but the time spent in them is not generally counted towards the 50 per cent of time that nursing students are expected to spend on practice placements.

The NMC indicated: 'We are looking specifically at what might be needed at the point of registration for a nurse in the 21st century. Currently we may well be putting nurses on the register who are not competent' (Duffin, 2005: 4). The possibility of incorporating a post-qualifying probationary year for newly qualified registrants is being considered. Yet another major review of pre-registration education is to be undertaken by the

NMC utilising a high-profile 'coalition' of the UK's four chief nursing officers, union leaders, directors of nursing and staff organisations (Duffin, 2005).

In response, university deans of nursing indicated that there was 'evidence that students on placements are under extreme pressure' (Duffin, 2005: 4). The NMC engages with nurse directors and Department of Health officials on how to improve placements, and give mentors 'protected time' for mentoring activities. The NMC, however, has no power to force trusts to introduce such measures but can recommend them, especially as there are major cost implications.

As just indicated, evaluation of mentoring activities is likely to highlight areas that are problematic or those that warrant further development. The mentor also has a duty to be up to date in all eight domains of the mentoring role. Thus, of necessity, the mentor has to engage in ongoing learning and continuing professional development in relation to mentoring and other roles or dimensions. So, what is continuing professional development and what is ongoing or lifelong learning?

## Continuing professional development for mentors

The ENB/DH (2001a) identifies practice educator and nurse lecturer as the next stages that the mentor can progress to if they wish to increase their teaching roles. The NMC (2006a) sees this progression as: registrant → mentor → practice teacher → qualified teacher. These can be intercalated between various education facilitator roles, such as clinical instructors and lecturer-practitioners.

From September 2008, an interim function will be introduced in the form of 'sign-off mentor', for which additional educational preparation is needed. These various stages can form part of the mentor's own ongoing professional development plans.

However, before moving on to these roles, the mentor needs to continue to develop mentoring knowledge and skills, and keep up to date with the latest developments related to the NMC's (2006a) competence and outcomes for mentors. They will have to attend annual updates, and most HEIs and trusts have a partnership agreement of ongoing development of their mentors. This constitutes a programme of learning for qualified mentors, which can incorporate e-learning mechanisms and reflective learning. Mentors who complete these programmes may be eligible for academic credit points. Furthermore, self-evaluation, along with personal research and clinical audits can highlight issues that can present opportunities for further development for mentors.

### Activity 8.7 – Mentor's annual updates

1. Following completion of a mentor preparation course, as a mentor you need to be aware of your own continuing professional development Consider how you can keep yourself up to date with new developments in professional knowledge and competence within your profession in relation to both clinical practice and mentoring. Discuss this with a colleague or your clinical supervisor.
2. What would the mentor expect to be covered in the annual update study day?

Mentor annual update events are usually one day long and are conducted by universities, where issues such as reliability can be raised, or better still, discussed in workshop groups. The NMC (2006a) makes some suggestions of activities to include on annual update study days. Some of the activities that can be explored include discussing inter- and intra-mentor reliability, and support mechanisms available for dealing with 'failing students'. New NMC rules and guidelines related to supporting learning and their implications can be explored. The NMC (2006a) also requires mentors to be subject to 'triennial reviews'. These include ascertaining during the DRP meeting (development review process) whether the mentor has engaged in mentoring activities, and kept them up to date.

### Mentoring RNs on specialist practice courses

Post-registration students on specialist programmes have specialist learning and assessment needs, a dimension which is not usually addressed on standard single-module mentor preparation courses. In the past, before the advent of mentoring courses subsequent to the Philips et al. (2000) study, teaching and assessing programmes were twice as long. For community nursing students, assessments were conducted by Community Practice Teachers (CPT) and Practice Work Teachers (PWT), the educational preparation for which being one academic year long. After the implementation of the novel mentor preparation course, whether mentors are at degree or masters level, it was soon realised that it wasn't sufficient to prepare them to assess the specific competencies of students on some specialist community courses (NMC, 2005d). The NMC (2006a) has therefore identified the practice teacher role as a role that mentors need to be educationally prepared for to mentor students on these courses, including those on SCPHN programmes.

As for the mentor's own ongoing professional development, a brief overview of what is continuing professional development and lifelong learning, along with relevant features of the mentor's leadership, follows.

Continuing professional development (CPD) is an inherent component of lifelong learning. It can be defined as 'a process of lifelong learning for all individuals and teams which meets the needs of patients and delivers the health outcomes and health care priorities of the NHS and which enables professionals to expand and fulfil their potential' (DoH, 1998: 42). At the practical level, Wallace (1999: 28) sees CPD as a 'term given to the learning which takes place in a professional's career after the point of qualification and/or registration'. Wallace prefers to see CPD as identified and intentional learning rather than learning that comes from the experience of professional practice.

The HPC (2006: 1) defines CPD as 'a range of learning activities through which health professionals maintain and develop throughout their career to make sure that they continue to be able to work safely, effectively and legally within their changing scope of practice'. CPD therefore reflects a responsible and proactive approach to one's own professional learning, and, as McGill and Beatty (1995) note, it involves an attitude to life and work that allows for creativity in one's professional activities.

The means and framework for CPD is further elaborated by Madden and Mitchell (1993) who suggest that organisations implement one of two main models of CPD: the sanction model and the benefit model. The employing or regulatory organisation that uses the sanction model tends to penalize the individual for not engaging in the necessary CPD. On the other hand, the organization utilising the benefit model does not threaten with sanctions but reinforces and, where possible, rewards individuals for voluntary CPD.

Alternatively, Wallace (1999) suggests the statutory, mandatory or permissive types of CPD. Statutory CPD is that which is undertaken as a result of statute or legislation. Mandatory CPD has a similar meaning, in that it is instigated by an official command or instruction by an authority and it is therefore compulsory. Wallace identifies the mandatory CPD model as one which suggests that CPD is a mandate by employers or regulatory bodies that has to be executed but no penalty is attached directly to it if not fulfilled. Permissive CPD is one in which the individual has choice.

Most healthcare professions or regulatory bodies have instituted some form of sanction or mandatory model of CPD. The NMC (2006g), for instance, indicates through post-registration education and practice (PREP) that every practising nurse, midwife or SCPHN must declare that they have undertaken a minimum of 35 hours of learning activity relevant to their practice during every three-year cycle to be able to re-register as a practitioner. The GMC and HPC have similar requirements.

The learning activity for meeting PREP requirements has to be in relevant areas of practice and can be in one or more of the key components of healthcare interventions aptly categorised in the *NHS KSF* (DoH, 2004b) as the six core dimensions. These are (1) communication, (2) personal and people development, (3) health, safety and security, (4) service improvement, (5) quality and (6) equality and diversity, as noted in Chapter 5, and apply to all NHS employees (except doctors, dentists and some board-level managers).

The *NHS KSF* also identifies 24 specific dimensions under *health and well-being, estates and facilities, information and knowledge* and *general*, that apply to some but not all jobs in the NHS. More specific details on each of these dimensions of healthcare interventions are presented in the *NHS KSF* document.

However, as the NMC only requires registrants to declare that they have engaged in the required amount of learning activity, PREP in itself does not constitute a guarantee of up-to-date clinical competence. There has been less research work on this in other professions. However, in nursing different researchers (e.g. Hunt, 1997) have previously indicated that nurses do not know about, understand or know how to use research findings.

The CPD advocated by the NMC is the minimum requirement for safe and competent practice, but it is recognised that the practitioner generally engages in substantially more learning than this minimum. Relevant university-based courses normally meet the NMC requirement adequately. However, self-directed or peer-based learning can also easily contribute to these requirements, as identified in the second outcome under evaluation of learning NMC domain (see Box 8.1). Self-directed is explained in detail in Chapter 2 under andragogy and the work of Knowles et al. (1998) and Rogers (2002). Peer learning is also well documented, in particular in the context of human and social capital (see for instance Gopee, 2002a).

*The mentor as a lifelong learner*
The concept of lifelong learning has been examined with intense attention in some quarters since the 1970s. The Department of Health (1998: 42) sees lifelong learning

as 'an investment in quality' and indicates that 'health professionals in all healthcare settings need the support of lifelong learning through continuing professional development programmes'.

## Activity 8.8 – Why lifelong learning?

List as many reasons as you can think of for healthcare professionals being required to be lifelong learners. How can healthcare professionals achieve lifelong learning? What are the probable problems with lifelong learning?

Lifelong learning differs from lifelong education in that while lifelong education refers to learning activities directed by established education institutions, and which normally leads to a qualification, lifelong learning refers to all forms of learning: formal, informal and incidental. The ENB (1994) indicated that nurses, midwives and health visitors who have developed as lifelong learners as a result of their pre-registration education have the following characteristics. They are:

- innovative in their practice;
- flexible to changing demand;
- resourceful in their methods of working;
- able to work as change agents;
- able to share good practice and knowledge;
- adaptable to changing health care needs;
- challenging and creative in their practice;
- self-reliant in their way of working;
- responsible and accountable for their work.

Extracted from a qualitative study of nurses' perceptions of lifelong learning, Gopee (2005) deduced a framework for the implementation of lifelong learning in healthcare, which comprises three groups of factors, namely:

- *Organisational factors* (e.g. time and release from work to attend CPD courses, work-based learning).
- *Socio-political factors* (e.g. social group influences in the clinical setting, clinical supervision).
- *Individual factors* (the healthcare professional's professionalism, learning as a natural human activity).

Furthermore, key NHS policy documents such as *NHS KSF* (DoH, 2004a), *Working Together – Learning Together: A Framework for Lifelong Learning for the NHS* (DoH, 2001b) and *Making a Difference* (DoH, 1999) all advocate the use of professional development plans (PDP) by all NHS healthcare professionals for their professional development throughout their careers. An example of a PDP slightly adapted from the *NHS KSF* is presented in Box 8.3

| Box 8.3   An example of a professional development plan |

Name: ................................   [Other relevant details e.g. clinical specialism]

| Relevant dimension | Learning and development activity | Hours and dates | Has the learning activity been (a) completed? (b) effective? | How will I apply this learning to my work? | Who else could I share this learning with? |
|---|---|---|---|---|---|
| 1. | | | | | |
| 2. | | | | | |
| 3. | | | | | |

The learning activity undertaken is of course also based on self-assessment. Consequently, every member of healthcare professions needs to be responsible for identifying their own learning needs. The NMC's *COPC* (2004a: clauses 3 and 4) states that 'as a registered nurse, midwife or health visitor, you are personally accountable for your practice and, in the exercise of your professional accountability, must "maintain and improve your professional knowledge and competence"; and "decline any duties and responsibilities unless able to perform them in a safe and skilled manner"'. This means that the healthcare registrants do not only have a responsibility to facilitate the learning of others, but also have a statutory responsibility to continue learning.

Thus healthcare professions explicitly encourage all trained staff to continue the process of learning, asking us to reflect and question the way we deliver care, and to engage in continuing development of our knowledge and skills.

## Chapter Summary

This chapter has focused on evaluation of mentoring, and, having completed this chapter, you will have learned:

- Why evaluate the effectiveness with which mentors facilitate learning and assessments, as well as other mentoring activities and roles.
- What evaluation is, the nature and various aspects of evaluation, and who evaluates the mentor's teaching activities.

- Different ways of evaluating clinically based and academically based teaching and assessment, and how mentors evaluate learning provision and assessments during practice placements. The use of models of evaluation, including heeding the findings of audits by external organisations such as the QAA and NMC.
- The likely problems of evaluation, the results of evaluations, issues arising from them, related consequences, and subsequent actions that can be taken.
- The opportunities and scope for ongoing learning arising from the results of evaluations, mentoring RNs on specialist practice courses, and continuing professional development in one's mentoring role and the mentor as a lifelong learner.

# Further Thoughts – a Journey Just Beginning

Mentoring is a career-long journey, whether it's to do with mentoring learners of one's own healthcare profession, or of allied health professions, medical students, or healthcare assistants. It is a journey that begins soon after your preceptee status ends. One of the strengths of nursing, midwifery and SCPHNs is the holistic approach that other healthcare professionals intend, endeavour and at times succeed in taking in their day-to-day practice. Some clinical settings have students all the time, others occasionally, but the actions that mentors take stay in the minds of healthcare professionals for several years, as they shape their careers and quality of patient care. The mentor's actions are therefore seminal in shaping the attitudes of practitioners for years to come.

On the other hand, as Rogers and Frieberg (1994: 375) indicate, 'not all journeys are trouble-free ... but the process alone makes us a bit wiser. Gaining wisdom comes not with time or age, but from living the challenges of life, learning from our mistakes, and building on experiences.' This book on mentoring was designed to achieve the objectives outlined in the introductory section, which is predominantly to examine the knowledge and understanding necessary for effective and mutually beneficial mentoring, and the NMC's (2006a) standards for mentors. The knowledge and skills acquired can be built on by pursuing the topic area further as a part of your own action plan. They could play a significant role along your career path, be it as a more senior clinical practitioner or in part- or full-time educational roles. What are the next steps you'd like to take when you have obtained your mentor qualification?

# References

Alaszwesski, K., Alaszwesski, H., Ayer, S., Manthorpe, M. and Walsh, M. (1998) *Risk Assessment and Management in Multi-agency, Multi-professional Health Care: Education and Practice (Research Highlights 34)*. London: ENB.

Anon (2006) 'Students press for £10,000 a year bursary', *Nursing Standard,* 20 (33): 6.

Argyle, M. (1994) *The Psychology of Interpersonal Behaviour* (5th edn). London: Penguin.

Ausubel, D., Novak, J. and Hanesian, H. (1978) *Educational Psychology: A Cognitive View*. New York: Rinehart & Winston.

Bahn, D. (2001) 'Social learning theory: its application in the context of nurse education', *Nurse Education Today,* 21 (2): 110–17.

Bandolier (1995) *Evidence-based Everything*. Available from: www.jr2.ox.ac.uk/bandolier/band12/b12-1.html. Accessed 20 February 2007.

Bandura, A. (1977) *Social Learning Theory*. Englewood Cliffs, NJ: Prentice-Hall.

Bandura, A. (1986) *Social Foundations of Thought and Action: A Social-cognitive Theory*. Englewood Cliffs, NJ: Prentice-Hall.

Barr, H. (2003) 'Interprofessional issues and work based learning', in J. Burton and N. Jackson (eds), *Work Based Learning in Primary Care*. Oxford: Radcliffe Medical.

Barr, H., Freeth, D., Hammick, M., Koppel, I. and Reeves, S. (2005) *The Evidence Base and Recommendations for Interprofessional Education in Health and Social Care*. Available from: http://www.swap.ac.uk/docs/learning/Evidence08.doc. (Accessed 5 January 2007).

Benner, P. (2001) *From Novice to Expert: Excellence and Power in Clinical Nursing Practice*. London: Addison-Wesley.

Berne, E. (1975) *What Do You Say After You Say Hello?* London: Corgi.

Binnie, A. and Titchen, A. (1999) *Freedom to Practice: The Development of Patient-centred Nursing*. Edinburgh: Butterworth-Heinemann.

Bloom, B. (1956) *Taxonomy of Educational Objectives: The Classification of Educational Goals, Handbook One: Cognitive Domain*. London: Longman.

Bondy, K.N. (1983) 'Criterion-referenced definitions for rating scales in clinical evaluation', *Journal of Nursing Education,* 22 (9): 376–82.

Boud, D. (1991) *Implementing Student Self-assessment (HERDSA Green Guide No 5)*. Australian Capital Territory, Australia: Higher Education Research and Development Society of Australasia.

Boud, D., Keogh, R. and Walker, D. (eds) (1985) *Reflection: Turning Experience into Learning*. London: Kogan Page.

Bowker, P., French, D., Atkin, S.L., Patmore, J.E., Walton, C. and Aye, M. (2005) 'Financing a diabetes network: care pathway based costing model for Type 1 diabetes mellitus', *Diabetic Medicine,* 23 (Suppl. 2): 107.

Bradshaw, A. (1997) 'Defining "competency" in nursing (part 1): a policy review', *Journal of Clinical Nursing,* 6 (5): 347–54.

British Association for Counselling and Psychotherapy (2006) *Supervision: Strategy and Action Plan*. Rugby: BACP.

Brown, I. (2005) 'Ethics in clinical education', in M. Rose and D. Best (eds), *Transforming Practice Through Clinical Education, Professional Supervision and Mentoring*. Edinburgh: Elsevier Churchill Livingstone.

Brown, J., Bullock, D. and Grossberg, S. (1999) 'How the basal ganglia use parallel excitatory and inhibitory learning pathways to selectively respond to unexpected rewarding cues', *Journal of Neuroscience,* 19 (23): 10502–11.

Brown, L. (editor-in-chief) (2002) *Shorter Oxford English Dictionary* (5th edn). Oxford: Oxford University Press.

Bruner, J. (1960) *The Process of Education.* Cambridge, MA: Harvard University Press.

Bryar, R.M. and Griffiths, J.M. (eds) (2003) *Practice Development in Community Nursing.* London: Arnold.

Burgoyne, J. and Reynolds, M. (eds) (1997) *Management Learning: Integrating Perspectives in Theory and Practice.* London: Sage.

Burnard, P. and Chapman, C. (1990) *Nurse Education: The Way Forward.* London: Scutari Press.

Carper, B. (1978) 'Fundamental patterns of knowing in nursing', *Advances in Nursing Science,* 1 (1): 13–23.

Castledine, G. (1998) *Writing, Documentation and Communication for Nurses.* Wiltshire: Mark Allen.

Centre for Advancement of Interprofessional Education (1997) *Interprofessional Education: A Definition Bulletin, 13:19.* London: CAIPE.

Chalmers, H., Swallow, V. and Miller, J. (2001) 'Accredited work-based learning: an approach for collaboration between higher education and practice', *Nurse Education Today,* 21 (8): 597–606.

Chartered Society for Physiotherapy (CSP) (2002) *Curriculum Framework for Qualifying Programmes in Physiotherapy.* Available from: www.csp.organisations.uk/uploads/docu-ments/CFforQSP.pdf. Accessed 14 June 2007.

Clarke, J.B. (1999) 'Evidence-based practice: a retrograde step? The importance of pluralism in evidence generation for the practice of healthcare', *Journal of Clinical Nursing,* 8 (1): 89–94.

Collinson, G. (2000) 'Encouraging the growth of the nurse entrepreneur', *Professional Nurse,* 15 (6): 365–7.

Cross, K.D. (1996) 'An analysis of the concept facilitation', *Nurse Education Today,* 16 (5): 350–5.

Curzon, L.B. (2001) *Teaching in Further Education* (5th edn). London: Continuum.

Dale, A.E. (2006) 'Determining guiding principles for evidence-based practice', *Nursing Standard,* 20 (25): 41–6.

Daloz, L.A. (1989) *Effective Teaching and Mentoring: Realizing the Transformational Power of Adult Learning Experiences.* San Francisco, CA: Jossey-Bass.

Darling, L.A.W. (1984) 'What do nurses want in a mentor?', *Journal of Nursing Administration,* 14 (10): 42–4.

Darling, L.A.W. (1985) 'What to do about toxic mentors?', *Journal of Nursing Administration,* 15 (5): 43–4.

Davies, I.K. (1982) *The Management of Learning* (2nd edn). New York: McGraw-Hill.

Davies, S. and Priestley, M.J. (2006) 'A reflective evaluation of patient handover practices', *Nursing Standard,* 20 (21): 49–52.

Dean, J. (2000) 'The nature and purpose of evaluation', in P. Nicklin and N. Kenworthy (eds), *Teaching and Assessing in Nursing Practice: An Experiential Approach.* London: Baillière Tindall.

Department of Health (DoH) (1990) *NHS and Community Care Act.* London: HMSO.

Department of Health (DoH) (1996) *Promoting Clinical Effectiveness: A Framework for Action in and through the NHS.* London: HMSO.

Department of Health (NHS Executive) (1998) *A First Class Service: Quality in the New NHS.* London: DoH.

Department of Health (DoH) (1999) *Making a Difference: Strengthening the Nursing, Midwifery and Health Visiting Contribution to Health and Health Care.* London: DoH.

Department of Health (DoH) (2001a) *Agenda for Change.* London: DoH.

Department of Health (DoH) (2001b) *Working Together – Learning Together: A Framework for Lifelong Learning for the NHS.* London: DoH.

Department of Health (DoH) (2002a) *Liberating the Talents: Helping Primary Care Trusts and Nurses to Deliver the NHS Plan.* Available from: http://www.doh.gov.uk/cno/liberatingtalents.htm. Accessed 14 June 2007.

Department of Health (DoH) (2002b) *PL CNO (2002) 5: Implementing the NHS Plan – Ten Key Roles for Nurses.* Available from: http://www.dh.gov.uk/PublicationsAndStatistics/LettersAndCirculars/ProfessionalLetters/ChiefNursingOfficerLetters. Accessed 14 June 2007.

Department of Health (DoH) (2004a) *NHS Knowledge and Skills Framework.* London: Stationery Office.

Department of Health (DoH) (2004b) *Patient Pathways: What Is a Patient Pathway?* Available from: www.dh.gov.uk/PolicyAndGuidance/OrganisationPolicy/Secondary Care/TreatmentCentre.html. Accessed 14 June 2007.

Department of Health (DoH) (2004c) *European Working Time Directive.* Available from: http://www. dh.gov.uk/Home/fs/en. Accessed 14 June 2007.

Department of Health (DoH) (2005) *Creating a Patient-led NHS: Delivering the NHS Improvement Plan.* London: DoH.

Department of Health (DoH) (2006a) *Common Learning in Health Professional Courses at Coventry University.* Available from: www.hss.coventry.ac.uk/firstwave. Accessed 14 June 2007.

Department of Health (DoH) (2006b) *Tackling Hospital Waiting: The 18-week Patient Pathway.* London: DoH.

Department of Health (DoH) (2006c) *Health Technology Assessment Programme.* London: DoH.

Department of Health (DoH) (2006d) *Modernising Nursing Careers: Setting the Direction.* Available from: http://195.33.102.76/assetRoot/04/13/87/57/04138757.pdf. Accessed 14 June 2007.

Department of Health (DoH) (2006e) *NHS Innovations: Annual Report 2004/5.* Available from: http://www.networks.nhs.uk/uploads/06/01/innovations_annual_report_0405.pdf. Accessed 14 June 2007.

Dewar, B.J. and Walker, E. (1999) 'Experiential learning: issues for supervision', *Journal of Advanced Nursing,* 30 (6): 1459–67.

Donabedian, A. (1988) 'The quality of care. How can it be assessed?', *American Journal of Public Health,* 260 (12): 1743.

Donaldson, I. (1992) 'The use of learning contracts in the clinical area', *Nurse Education Today,* 12 (6): 431–6.

Donaldson, J.H. and Carter, D. (2005) 'The value of role modelling: perceptions of undergraduate and diploma nursing (adult) students', *Nurse Education in Practice,* 5 (6): 353–9.

Dougherty, L. and Lister, S. (eds) (2006) *The Royal Marsden Hospital Manual of Clinical Nursing Procedures* (7th edn). Oxford: Blackwell.

Dreyfus, S.E. and Dreyfus, H.L. (1980) *A Five-stage Model of the Mental Activities involved in Directed Skill Acquisition.* Unpublished report supported by the Air Force Office of Scientific Research (USA). Berkeley, CA: University of California.

Duffin, C. (2005) 'Pre-registration education to undergo major review', *Nursing Standard,* 19 (26): 4.

Duffy, K. (2004) *Mentors Need to Learn to Fail Students*. Available from: www.nmc-uk.org. Accessed 14 June 2007.

Egan, G. (2002) *The Skilled Helper: A Problem-management and Opportunity-development Approach to Helping*. Pacific Grove, CA: Brooks/Cole.

English National Board for Nursing, Midwifery and Health Visiting (ENB) (1987) *Management of Change in Nurse Education*. London: ENB.

English National Board for Nursing, Midwifery and Health Visiting (ENB) (1994) *Creating Lifelong Learners*. London: ENB.

English National Board for Nursing, Midwifery and Health Visiting (ENB) (1995) *Regulations and Guidelines for the Approval of Institutions and Courses*. London: ENB.

English National Board for Nursing, Midwifery and Health Visiting (ENB) (1997) *Standards for Approval of Higher Education Institutions and Programmes*. London: ENB.

English National Board for Nursing, Midwifery and Health Visiting (ENB) and Department of Health (2001a) *Preparation of Mentors and Teachers: A New Framework*. London: ENB.

English National Board for Nursing, Midwifery and Health Visiting (ENB) and Department of Health (2001b) *Placements in focus*. London: ENB.

Entwistle, N. (1994) *Supporting Effective Learning: A Research Perspective*. Edinburgh: University of Edinburgh.

Evans, D. (2003) 'Hierarchy of evidence: a framework for ranking evidence evaluating healthcare interventions', *Journal of Clinical Nursing*, 12 (1): 77–84.

Falchikov, N. (1986) 'Product comparisons and process benefits of collaborative peer group and self assessment', *Assessment and Evaluation in Higher Education*, 11 (2): 146–66.

Faugier, J. (2005a) 'Reality check', *Nursing Standard*, 19 (19): 14–15.

Faugier, J. (2005b) 'Developing a new generation of nurse entrepreneurs', *Nursing Standard*, 19 (30): 49–53.

Field, J. (1999) 'Participation under the magnifying glass', *Adults Learning*, 11 (3): 10–13.

Fitts, P.M. and Posner, M.I. (1973) *Human Performance*. London: Prentice-Hall.

Flanagan, J., Baldwin, S. and Clarke, D. (2000) 'Work-based learning as a means of developing and assessing nursing competence', *Journal of Clinical Nursing*, 9 (3): 360–8.

Freeth, D. and Nicol, M. (1998) 'Learning clinical skills: an interprofessional approach', *Nurse Education Today*, 18 (6): 455–61.

Freeth, D., Reeves, S., Koppel, I., Hammick, M. and Barr, H. (2005) *Evaluating Interprofessional Education: A Self-help Guide Occasional Paper No 5*. London: Higher Education Academy.

Freire, P. (1996) *Pedagogy of the Oppressed*. London: Penguin.

Fretwell, J.E. (1980) 'An inquiry into the ward learning environment', *Nursing Times*, 26 June.

Furlong, J. and Maynard, T. (1995) *Mentoring Student Teachers*. London: Routledge.

Gagné, R. (1983) *The Conditions of Learning and Theory of Instruction* (4th edn). New York: Holt, Rinehart & Winston.

Gallagher, A. and Wainwright, P. (2005) 'The ethical divide', *Nursing Standard*, 20 (7): 22–5.

Garbett, R. and McCormack, B. (2002) 'A concept analysis of practice development', *NTresearch*, 7 (2): 87–100.

Ghazi, F. and Henshaw, L. (1998) 'How to keep student nurses motivated', *Nursing Standard*, 13 (8): 43–8.

Gibbs, G. (1988) *Improving the Quality of Student Learning*. Bristol: Technical Education Services.

Girot, E. (1993) 'Assessment of competence in clinical practice: a review of literature', *Nurse Education Today*, 13 (2): 83–90.

Gopee, N. (2000) 'Self-assessment and the concept of the lifelong learning nurse', *British Journal of Nursing*, 9 (11): 724–9.

Gopee, N. (2001) 'The role of peer assessment and peer review in nursing', *British Journal of Nursing*, 10 (2): 115–21.

Gopee, N. (2002a) 'Human and social capital as facilitators of lifelong learning in nursing', *Nurse Education Today,* 22 (8): 608–16.

Gopee, N. (2002b) 'Demonstrating critical analysis in academic assignments', *Nursing Standard,* 16 (35): 45–52.

Gopee, N. (2005) 'Facilitating the implementation of lifelong learning in nursing', *British Journal of Nursing,* 14 (14): 761–7.

Gopee, N., Tyrell, A., Raven, S., Thomas, K. and Hari, T. (2004) 'Effective clinical learning in primary care settings', *Nursing Standard,* 18 (37): 33–7.

Gray, J.A.M. (2001) *Evidence-based Health Care: How to Make Policy and Management Decisions* (2nd edn). Edinburgh: Churchill Livingstone.

Greenhalgh, T. (1997) *How to Read a Paper.* London: BMJ.

Guba, E.G. and Lincoln, Y.S. (1989) *Fourth Generation Evaluation.* London: Sage.

Guile, D. and Young, M. (1996) 'Further professional development and further education teachers: setting a new agenda for work-based learning', in I. Woodward (ed.), *Continuing Professional Development: Issues in Design and Delivery.* London: Cassell.

Handy, C. (1989) *Age of Unreason.* London: Business Books.

Hargreaves, J. (1996) 'Credit where credit's due: work-based learning in professional practice', *Journal of Clinical Nursing,* 5 (2): 165–9.

Harrison, S. (2005) 'Closing the poverty trap between study and work [Analysis]', *Nursing Standard,* 19 (40): 15–16.

Hawkins, P. and Shohet, R. (2006) *Supervision in the Helping Professions* (3rd edn). Milton Keynes: Open University Press.

Health Professions Council (HPC) (2006) *Your Guide to our Standards for Continuing Professional Education.* London: HPC.

Health Professions Council (HPC) (2007) *What Is the HPC?* Available from: http://www.hpc-uk.org/aboutus/intro/. Accessed 22 January 2007.

Hean, S., Clark, J.M., Adams, K., Humphris, D. and Lathlean, J. (2006) 'Being seen by others as we see ourselves: the congruence between the in-group and outgroup perceptions of health and social care students', *Learning in Health and Social Care,* 5 (1): 10–22.

Heirs, B. and Farrell, P. (1986) *The Professional Decision Thinker.* London: Sidgwick & Jackson.

Henderson, A., Twentyman, M., Heel, A. and Lloyd, B. (2006) 'Students' perception of the psychosocial clinical learning environment: An evaluation of placement models', *Nurse Education Today,* 26 (7): 564–71.

Heron, J. (1989) *Six Category Intervention Analysis: Human Potential Research Project* (2nd edn). Guildford: University of Surrey.

Higher Education Academy (HEA) (2005) *Occasional Paper 6: Making Practice-based Learning Work.* London: HEA.

Honey, P. and Mumford, A. (2000) *The Learning Styles Helper's Guide.* Maidenhead: Peter Honey.

Hughes, C. (1999) 'The dire in self-directed learning', *Adults Learning,* 11 (2): 7–9.

Hughes, L. and Marsh, T. (2006) *Planning for an Interprofessional Workforce.* Creating an Interprofessional Workforce (CIPW) Programme. Available from: www.dh.gov.uk/PolicyAndGuidance. Accessed 25 May 2006.

Hunt, J. (1981) 'Indicators of nursing practice: the use of nursing research findings', *Journal of Advanced Nursing,* 6 (3): 189–94.

Hunt, J. (1997) 'Towards evidence-based practice', *Nursing Management,* 4 (2): 14–17.

Hutchings, A. and Sanders, L. (2001) 'Developing a learning pathway for student nurses', *Nursing Standard,* 15 (40): 38–41.

Issakidis, C. and Andrews, G. (2006) 'Who treats whom? An application of the Pathways to Care model in Australia', *Australian & New Zealand Journal of Psychiatry,* 40 (1): 74–86.

Jarvis, P. (1995) *Adult and Continuing Education.* London: Croom Helm.

Jarvis, P. and Gibson, S. (1997) *The Teacher Practitioner and Mentor* (2nd edn). Cheltenham: Stanley Thornes.

Jeffs, T. (2003) 'Quest for knowledge begins with a recognition of shared ignorance', *Adults Learning,* 14 (6): 28.

Joyce, B., Calhoun, E. and Hopkins, D. (2002) *Models of Learning: Tools for Teaching (2nd edn)*. Buckingham: Open University Press.

Kendall-Raynor, P. (2007) 'Nurse cleared in supervision case is to face NMC', *Nursing Standard,* 21 (17): 9.

Kerry, T. and Mayes, A.S. (eds) (1995) *Issues in Mentoring.* London: Routledge and The Open University.

Knowles, M. (1990) *The Adult Learner: A Neglected Species* (4th edn). Houston, TX: Gulf Publishing.

Knowles, M., Holton III, E.F. and Swanson, R.A. (1998) *The Adult Learner* (5th edn). Woburn (USA), Butterworth-Heinemann.

Kohler, W. (1925) 'The mentality of apes'. In E. Smith, S. Nolen-Hoeksema and B. Fredrickson (eds) (2003), *Atkinson and Hilgard's Introduction to Psychology* (14th edn). London: Thomson/Wadsworth.

Kolb, D. (1984) *Experiential Learning: Experience as the Source of Learning and Development.* London: Prentice-Hall.

Kopp, P. (2001) 'Fit for practice – 6.1: What is evidence-based practice?', *Nursing Times,* 97 (22): 47–50.

Kouzes, J.M. and Posner, B.Z. (2003) *The Leadership Challenge.* San Francisco, CA: Jossey-Bass.

Kramer, M. (1974) *Reality Shock: Why Nurses Leave Nursing.* St. Louis, MO: Mosby.

Krathwohl, D.R. (2002) A revision of Blooms Taxonomy: An overview', *Theory into practice,* 41 (4): 212–18.

Krathwohl, D., Bloom, B. and Masia, B. (1964) *A Taxonomy of Educational Objectives: The Classification of Education Goals, Handbook 2: Affective Domain.* New York: McKay.

Lang, N. (1976) *Issues in Quality Assurance in Nursing: ANA Issues in Evaluative Research.* Kansas City: American Nursing Association.

Lankshear, A. (1990) 'Failure to fail: the teacher's dilemma', *Nursing Standard,* 4 (20): 35–7.

Lewin, K. (1951) *Field Theory in Social Science.* London: Harper & Row.

Liefer, D. (2005) 'My practice: government policy changes allowed an entrepreneurial nurse to pave the way for nurse-led general practices', *Nursing Standard,* 19 (22): 58.

Lindberg, J.B., Hunter, M.L. and Kruszewski, A.Z. (1998) *Introduction to Nursing: Concepts, Issues and Opportunities* (3rd edn). Philadelphia, PA: Lippincott.

Lloyd, N. (1999) 'BJTR and interdisciplinary practice: moving forward', *British Journal of Therapy and Rehabilitation,* 6 (12): 573.

Long, A., Kneafsey, R., Ryan, J. and Howard, J. (2001) *Exploring the Role and Contribution of the Nurse in the Multi-professional Rehabilitation Team (Research Highlights 45).* London: ENB.

Lunyk-Child, O.L., Crooks, D., Ellis, P.J., Ofosu, C., O'Mara, L. and Rideout, E. (2001) 'Self-directed learning: faculty and student perceptions', *Journal of Nursing Education,* 40 (3): 116–23.

McCaughan, D. (1999) 'Developing critical appraisal skills', *Professional Nurse,* 14 (12): 843–7.

McCaughan, D., Thompson, C., Cullum, N., Sheldon, T.A. and Thompson, D.R. (2002) 'Acute care: nurses' perceptions of barriers to using research information in clinical decision-making', *Journal of Advanced Nursing,* 39 (1): 46–60.

McCormack, B., Manley, K., Kitson, A., Titchen, A. and Harvey, G. (1999) 'Towards practice development – a vision in reality or a reality without vision?', *Journal of Nursing Management,* 7 (5): 255–64.

McGill, I. and Beatty, L. (1995/1998) 'Continuing Professional Development', in C.M. Downie and P. Basford (eds), *Teaching and Assessing in Clinical Practice.* London: University of Greenwich.

McGivney, V. (2003) *Adult Learning Pathways: Through Routes or Cul-de-sac*. Leicester: NIACE.

McGregor, D. (1987) *The Human Side of Enterprise*. London: Penguin.

McKenna, H.P. (1995) 'Dissemination and application of mental health nursing research', *British Journal of Nursing*, 4 (21): 1257–63.

McNicholl, M.P., Dunne, K., Garvey, A., Sharkey, R. and Bradley, A. (2006) 'Using the Liverpool care pathway for a dying patient', *Nursing Standard*, 20 (38): 46–50.

Madden, C. and Mitchell, V. (1993) *Professions, Standards and Competence: A Survey of Continuing Education for the Professions*. Bristol: Department for Continuing Education, University of Bristol.

Mallik, M. and McGowan, B. (2006) 'Issues in practice-based learning in nursing in the United Kingdom and the Republic of Ireland: results from a multiprofessional scoping exercise', *Nurse Education Today*, 27 (1): 52–9.

Marton, F., Hounsell, D. and Entwistle, N. (eds) (1997) *The Experience of Learning* (2nd edn). Edinburgh: Scottish Academic Press.

Maslow, A.H. (1987) *Motivation and Personality* (3rd edn). London: Harper & Row.

Maxwell, R.J. (1984) 'Quality assurance in health care', *British Medical Journal*, 288 (6428): 1470–2.

Mazhindu, G.N. (1990) 'Contract learning reconsidered: a critical examination of implications for application in nurse education', *Journal of Advanced Nursing*, 15 (1): 101–9.

Mezirow, J. (1983) 'A critical theory of adult learning and education', in M. Tight (ed.), *Adult Learning and Education*. London: Croom Helm.

Mikkelsen Kyrkjebø, J. and Hage, I. (2005) 'What we know and what they do: nursing students' experiences of improvement knowledge in clinical practice', *Nurse Education Today*, 25 (3): 167–75.

Miller, C., Ross, N. and Freeman, M. (1999) *The Role of Collaborative/Shared Learning in Pre- and Post-Registration Education in Nursing, Midwifery and Health Visiting (Research Highlights 39)*. London: ENB.

Morrison, S., Boohan, M., Moutray, M. and Jenkins, J. (2004) 'Developing pre-qualification interprofessional education', *Nurse Education in Practice*, 4 (1): 20–9.

Morton-Cooper, A. and Wilkes, J. (1993) 'What is teaching?', *Nursing Times*, 89 (41): i–viii.

Mulholland, J., Scammell, J., Turnock, C. and Gregg, B. (2006) *Making Practice-based Learning Work: Final Report*. Northumbria: Northumbria University.

Mullins, L. (2005) *Management and Organizational Behaviour* (7th edn). London: Pitman.

National Committee of Inquiry into Higher Education (1997) *Higher Education in the Learning Society (The Dearing Report)*. Norwich: HMSO.

Neary, M. (2000a) *Teaching, Assessing and Evaluation for Clinical Competence*. Cheltenham: Stanley Thornes.

Neary, M. (2000b) 'Responsive assessment of clinical competence (Part 1)', *Nursing Standard*, 15 (9): 34–6.

NHS Institute for Innovation and Improvement (2007) *About the Institute*. Available from: www.institute.nhs.uk. Accessed 29 January 2007.

Nicklin, P. and Kenworthy, N. (eds) (2000) *Teaching and Assessing in Nursing Practice: An Experiential Approach* (3rd edn). London: Baillière Tindall.

Northcott, N. (1989) 'Planning the transition from student to staff nurse', *Senior Nurse*, 9 (7): 27–8.

Nursing and Midwifery Council (NMC) (2004a) *The NMC Code of Professional Conduct: Standards for Conduct, Performance and Ethics*. London: NMC.

Nursing and Midwifery Council (NMC) (2004b) *Standards of Proficiency for Pre-registration Nursing Education*. London: NMC.

Nursing and Midwifery Council (NMC) (2004c) *Reporting Unfitness to Practise: A Guide for Employers and Managers*. London: NMC.

Nursing and Midwifery Council (NMC) (2004d) *Standards of Proficiency for Specialist Community Public Health Nurses.* London: NMC.

Nursing and Midwifery Council (NMC) (2005a) *Guidelines for Records and Record-keeping.* London: NMC.

Nursing and Midwifery Council (NMC) (2005b) *NMC Consultation on Proposals Arising from a Review of Fitness for Practice at the Point of Registration.* London: NMC.

Nursing and Midwifery Council (NMC) (2006a) *A Standard to Support Learning and Assessment in Practice.* London: NMC.

Nursing and Midwifery Council (NMC) (2006b) *Preceptorship A–Z Advice Sheet.* Available from: www.nmc-uk.org. Accessed 14 June 2007.

Nursing and Midwifery Council (NMC) (2006c) *Preceptorship Guidelines.* NMC Circular 21/2006. Available from: www.nmc-uk.org. Accessed 14 June 2007.

Nursing and Midwifery Council (NMC) (2006d) *Responses to the NMC Consultation on Proposals Arising from a Review of Fitness for Practice at the Point of Registration. Final Report.* London: NMC.

Nursing and Midwifery Council (NMC) (2006e) *Advance Information to Programme Providers Regarding the NMC's Intention to Introduce Essential Skills Clusters for Pre-registrants Nursing Programmes. NMC Circular 35/2006.* Available from: www.nmc-uk.org. Accessed 14 June 2007.

Nursing and Midwifery Council (NMC) (2006f) *UK-wide Quality Assurance Framework.* Available from: www.nmc-uk.org. Accessed 14 June 2007.

Nursing and Midwifery Council (NMC) (2006g) *The PREP Handbook.* Available from: www.nmc-uk.org. Accessed 14 June 2007.

Nursing and Midwifery Council (NMC) (2007) *The New Draft Code of Conduct.* Available from: www.nmc-uk.org. Accessed 14 June 2007.

Open University (1984) *A Systematic Approach to Nursing Care.* Milton Keynes: Open University Press.

Open University (2001) *Assessing Practice in Nursing and Midwifery – K320 Workbook 3.* Milton Keynes: Open University Press.

Orton, H. (1981) 'Ward learning climate and student nurse response', *Nursing Times,* 4 June.

Orton, H.D., Prowse, J. and Millen, C. (1993) *Charting the Way to Excellence (Ward Learning Climate Project).* Sheffield: Sheffield Hallam University.

Overill, S. (1998) 'A practical guide to care pathways', *Journal of Integrated Care,* 2: 93–8.

Page, S. (2001) 'Demystifying practice development', *Nursing Times,* 97 (22): 36–7.

Palfreyman, S., Tod, A. and Doyle, J. (2003) 'Comparing evidence-based practice of nurses and physiotherapists', *British Journal of Nursing,* 12 (4): 246–53.

Peters, R.S. (1966) *Ethics and Education.* London: George Allen & Unwin.

Peters, R.S. (1973) *The Philosophy of Education (Oxford Readings in Philosophy).* Oxford: Oxford University Press.

Phillips, T., Schostak, J. and Tyler, J. (2000) *Practice and Assessment in Nursing and Midwifery: Doing it for Real (Researching Professional Education).* London: ENB.

Piaget, J. (1962) 'The stages of intellectual development of the child', in I. Roth (ed.), *Introduction to Psychology.* Milton Keynes: LEA & Open University.

Pirrie, A., Wilson, V., Harden, R.M. and Elsegood, J. (1998) 'Multiprofessional Education: part two – promoting cohesive practice in healthcare (AMEE Guide No 12)', *Medical Teacher,* 20 (5): 409–16.

Polanyi, M. (1958) *Personal Knowledge.* London: Routledge.

Pollard, C. and Hibbert, C. (2004) 'Expanding student learning using patient pathways', *Nursing Standard,* 19 (2): 40–3.

Proctor, B. (2001) 'Training for the supervision alliance: attitude, skills and intention', in J. Cutcliffe, T. Butterworth and B. Proctor (eds), *Fundamental Themes in Clinical Supervision.* London: Routledge.

Quality Assurance Agency for Higher Education (QAA) (2001) *Code of Practice for the Assurance of Academic Quality and Standards in Higher Education. Section 9: Placement Learning*, Gloucester: QAA.

Quinn, F.M. and Hughes, S.J. (2007) *Quinn's Principles and Practice of Nurse Education* (5th edn). Cheltenham: Nelson Thornes.

Ramsden, P. (ed.) (1988) *Improving Learning: New Perspectives*. London: Kogan Page.

Rattray, J.E., Paul, F. and Tully, V. (2006) 'Partnership working between a higher education institution and NHS Trusts: developing an acute and critical care module', *Nursing in Critical Care*, 11 (3): 111–17.

Redfern, S. (1998) 'Evaluation: drawing comparisons or achieving consensus?', *NTresearch*, 3 (6): 464–74.

Reeves, S. and Pryce, A. (1998) 'Emerging themes: an exploratory research project of an interprofessional education module for medical, dental and nursing students', *Nurse Education Today*, 18 (7): 534–41.

Roberts, P., Priest, H. and Bromage, C. (2001) 'Selecting and utilising data sources to evaluate health care education', *Nurse Researcher*, 8 (3): 15–29.

Rogers, A. (2002) *Teaching Adults* (3rd edn). Buckingham: Open University Press.

Rogers, C. (1983) *Freedom to Learn in the 80s.* Ohio: Charles Merrill.

Rogers, C. and Freiberg, H.J. (1994) *Freedom to Learn* (3rd edn). New Jersey: Pearson Education.

Rogers, E. and Shoemaker, F. (1971) *Communication of Innovations: A Cross-cultural Report* (2nd edn). New York: Free Press.

Rolfe, G. (1999) 'Insufficient evidence: the problems of evidence-based nursing', *Nurse Education Today,* 19 (6): 433–42.

Rotem, A. and Hart, G. (1995) 'The clinical learning environment: nurses' perceptions of professional development in clinical settings', *Nurse Education Today*, 15 (1): 3–10.

Rowntree, D. (1987) *Assessing Students: How Shall We Know Them?* London: Kogan Page.

Royal College of Nursing (RCN) (1996) *The Royal College of Nursing Clinical Effectiveness Initiative: A Strategic Framework.* London: RCN.

Royal College of Nursing (RCN) (2002) *Helping Students Get the Best from Their Practice Placements (A Royal College of Nursing Toolkit).* London: RCN.

Royal College of Nursing (RCN) (2003) *Quality Education for Quality Care: A Position Statement for Nursing Education.* London: RCN.

Royal College of Nursing (RCN) (2004) *The Future Nurse: Evidence of the Impact of Registered Nurses.* London: RCN.

Royal College of Nursing (RCN) (2005a) *Guidance for Mentors of Student Nurses and Midwives: A RCN Toolkit.* London: RCN.

Royal College of Nursing (RCN) (2005b) *Maxi Nurses: Nurses Working in Advanced and Extended Roles Promoting and Developing Patient-centred Healthcare.* London: RCN.

Royal College of Nursing (RCN) (2006) *Practice Development.* London: RCN.

Rycroft-Malone, J., Harvey, G., Kitson, A., McCormack, B., Seers, K. and Titchen, A. (2002) 'Getting evidence into practice', *Nursing Standard*, 16 (37): 38–43.

Sackett, D.L., Strauss, S.E., Richardson, S.W., Rosenburg, W. and Haynes, R.B. (2000) *Evidence-based Medicine: How to Practice and Teach EBM* (2nd edn). Edinburgh: Churchill Livingstone.

Sackett, D.L., Rosenburg, W., Gray, J.M., Haynes, R.B. and Richardson, S.W. (1996) 'Evidence-based medicine: what it is and what it isn't', *BMJ*, 312 (7023): 71–2.

Salmon, D. and Jones, M. (2001) 'Shaping the interprofessional agenda: a study examining qualified nurses' perceptions of learning with each other', *Nurse Education Today*, 21 (1): 18–25.

Satterly, D. (1981) *Assessment in Schools: Theory and Practice in Education*. Oxford: Blackwell Science.

Scammell, B. (1990) *Communication Skills*. Basingstoke: Macmillan.

Scheler, M. (1980) *Problems of Sociology of Knowledge*. London: Routledge & Kegan Paul.

Schon, D. (1995) *The Reflective Practitioner: How Professionals Think in Action*. Aldershot: Arena.

Scullion, P. (2002) 'Effective dissemination strategies', *Nurse Researcher. Qualitative Approaches,* 10 (1): 65–7.

Shardlow, S. and Doel, M. (1996) *Practice Learning and Teaching*. London: British Association of Social Workers/Macmillan.

Simpson, J. and Weiner, E. (1989) *The Oxford English Dictionary* (2nd edn). Oxford: Oxford University Press.

Sines, D., Harris, D., Firth, J. and Boden, L. (2006) 'Applied leadership: ensuring fitness for practice', *Nursing Management,* 13 (8): 28–31.

Skinner, B.F. (1971) *Beyond Freedom and Dignity*. New York: Alfred Knopf.

Sleep, J. and Clark, E. (1999) 'Weighing up the evidence: the contribution of critical literature reviews to the development of practice', *NTresearch,* 4 (1): 306–13.

Spouse, J. (2001a) 'Bridging theory and practice in the supervisory relationship: a sociocultural perspective', *Journal of Advanced Nursing,* 33 (4): 512–22.

Spouse, J. (2001b) 'Work-based learning in healthcare environments', *Nurse Education in Practice,* 1 (1): 12–18.

Steinaker, N.W. and Bell, M.R. (1979) *The Experiential Learning: A New Approach to Teaching and Learning*. New York: Academic Press.

Stuart, C.C. (2007) *Assessment, Supervision and Support in Clinical Practice* (2nd edn). Edinburgh: Churchill Livingstone.

Sullivan, E.J. and Decker, P.J. (2005) *Effective Leadership and Management in Nursing*. Upper Saddle River, NJ: Pearson/Prentice-Hall International.

Thiroux, J. and Krasemann, K. (2007) *Ethics, Theory and Practice* (9th edn). Upper Saddle River, NJ: Pearson/Prentice-Hall.

Thomas, L. (2005) 'An inspiration to all', *Nursing Standard,* 19 (24): 27.

Thompson, C. (1998) 'Testing our intuition', *Nursing Standard,* 12 (27): 18.

Thompson, C., McCaughan, D., Cullum, N., Sheldon, T. and Raynor, P. (2002) 'The value of research in clinical decision-making', *Nursing Times,* 98 (42): 30–4.

Titchen, A. (2003) 'The practice development diamond', paper presented at the 2003 International Nursing Research Conference, London.

UNISON (2006) *Learning the Hard Way*. London: UNISON.

United Kingdom Central Council for Nursing, Midwifery and Health Visiting (UKCC) (1999) *Fitness for Practice*. London: UKCC.

United Kingdom Central Council for Nursing, Midwifery and Health Visiting (UKCC) (2000) *The Scope of Professional Practice: A Study of Its Implementation*. London: UKCC.

Unsworth, J. (2000) 'Practice development: a concept analysis', *Journal of Nursing Management,* 8 (6): 317–26.

van Eps, M., Cooke, M., Creedy, D. and Walker, R. (2006) Student evaluations of a year-long mentorship program: A quality improvement initiative. *Nurse Education Today,* 26 (6): 519–24.

van Wijngaarden, J.D.H., Dirks, M., Dippel, D.W.J., Minkman, M. and Niessen, L.W. (2006) 'Towards effective and efficient care pathways: thrombolysis in acute ischaemic stroke' *Qjm,* 99 (4): 267–72.

Waddington, K. and Marsh, L. (1998) 'Work-based learning in a multigrade, multiskilled group: an action research perspective', *Managing Clinical Nursing,* 2 (4): 101–4.

Wallace, M. (1999) *Lifelong Learning: PREP in Action.* Edinburgh: Churchill Livingstone.

Walsh, M. and Ford, P. (1989) *Nursing Rituals, Research and Rational Actions.* Oxford: Heinemann Nursing.

Ward, C. and McCormack, B. (2000) 'Creating an adult learning culture through practice development', *Nurse Education Today,* 20 (4): 259–66.

Watkins, K. and Marsick, V. (1992) 'Building the learning organisation: a new role for human resource developers', *Studies in Continuing Education,* 14 (2): 115–29.

Watson, J.B. (1978) 'The great psychologists: from Aristotle to Freud', in E. Smith, S. Nolen-Hoeksema and B. Fredrickson (eds) (2003), *Atkinson and Hilgard's Introduction to Psychology* (14th edn). London: Thomson/Wadsworth.

West Midlands South Strategic Health Authority (2006) *Multi-professional Practice Environment Profile.* Coventry: Coventry University.

White, E., Davies, S., Twinn, S. and Rilet, E. (1993) *A Detailed Study of the Relationship between Teaching, Support, Supervision, and Role Modelling for Students in Clinical Areas within the Context of Project 2000 Courses (Research Highlight 3).* London: ENB.

Wilson, V., Pirrie, A. and Finnigan, J. (1998) 'Encouraging learning: a study of continuing professional development in health care', *Health Bulletin,* 56 (3): 667–74.

Wood, S. (2005) 'The experiences of a group of pre-registration mental health nursing students', *Nurse Education Today,* 25 (3): 189–96.

Wright, S. (1990) *Building and Using a Model of Nursing.* London: Edward Arnold.

# Index